when in doubt, see the patient

*Travels through the Landscapes
of American Health Care*

By Norbert Voelkel, MD

ISBN: 0615741266
ISBN 13: 9780615741260

Table of Contents

When in Doubt, See the Patient

"We accepted, so to speak, a second Bill of Rights under which a new basis of security and prosperity can be established for all regardless of the station, race, or creed. Among these are…the right to adequate medical care and the opportunity to achieve and enjoy good health."

F.D. Roosevelt, January 11, 1944

"When Americans began looking upon rights as some sort of positive duty on others to provide them with certain things, that was when the quality of health care in America began plummeting. That was what Medicare and Medicaid were all about—the so-called right of poor people and the elderly to health care. It is not a coincidence that what began as the finest health care system in the world had turned into a system that is now in perpetual crisis."

Jacob G. Hornberger, 2009
Founder of the Future of Freedom Foundation

"My fellow Americans: American health care industry is an industry like any other industry."

Ronald. Reagan

"The health care industry or medical industry is a sector within the economic system that provides goods and services to treat patients with curative, preventative, rehabilitative, palliative, or, at times, unnecessary care."

United States Department of Labor, 2007

1

"No American should ever have to fear being left uncared for in the middle of the world's most advanced health care system."

Mitt Romney, 2012

"Supporters and detractors alike refer to the law (the Affordable Care Act) as Obamacare. I don't mind because I do care. And because of Obamacare, we are moving forward a health care system that broadly provides health security."

Barack Obama, 2012

"Universal coverage—one health care nation under God."

Anonymous

Introduction

As the first Baby Boomers begin to retire, the aging of America will increasingly become an enormous health care problem, quickly followed by the mounting epidemic of obesity. America will need more doctors. The Virginia Commonwealth University is finishing the construction of a new medical school building and increased its 2013 first-year class size to two hundred students, while Stanford University will continue to accept only eighty medical students. A gigantic health care industry, with annual costs at $2.6 trillion in 2010, is torn between the extremes of cookie-cutter, guideline-driven medical care and highly personalized treatment strategies. The Affordable Care Act (ACA) was in front of Supreme Court judges and pharmaceutical companies continued to interrupt the daily evening news on television with advertisements that promote their purple or green COPD inhaled drug products and promise benefits from the use of their antidepressants and pills that treat erectile dysfunction. As the Boomers now experience for themselves that aging is not for wimps, they face the prospect of their own illnesses and recognize that they will be able to afford perhaps diabetes and hypertension but not breast cancer or leukemia.

The Boomers will need a map to find their way around when they navigate through the health care system. This reality has been recognized by two Washington University (St. Louis) medical students, Nathan Moore and Elisabeth Askin, who recently published their *Health Care Handbook*[1] a clear and concise guide to the United States health care system. The reputable, internationally read, and widely quoted *New England Journal of Medicine* (*NEJM*), which celebrated its 200th anniversary in 2012, has become an important forum for discussions of American health care delivery problems, like the issues of electronic health records, access to health care, health care policies, and reimbursement plans. The *Journal* gives a voice to the ever-increasing number of health care regulation analysts. These experts are academically trained and often work for health information companies. They dissect business models, the enormous influence of insurance carriers, and the expectations of health care consumers. They propose new metrics for the quality of health care, and they rarely compare American health care with the health care delivered in other countries and by other provider models.

What has become noticeable, and remarkably has not become a subject of expert analysis, is the new vocabulary and syntax used to describe American health care. The new health care language and the use and abuse of omnipresent and omniscient flat screens are both equally responsible for my wanting to write this small book. Like most bilinguals, my ear is tuned to the new words and sensitive to hidden agendas and assumptions that are the undercurrents and sinkholes that the use of this language attempts to hide. Terms like "productivity paradox," "specialized environments for caregivers," and "uncompensated care costs" are recent blooms of this plant. Surely, a new sub-sub-specialty group of experts can now begin to investigate the exciting new field termed "health care semantics." They will explain the meaning of "non-urgent triage desks" and of "prudent layperson" language to all of us.

There is now some discussion of the role of information technology (IT) systems and their increasingly demanding presence in modern medicine. The health care industry evolution has been driven largely by computers and flat screens, and health care providers all over the world spend more and more of their time entering data and documenting their caregiving efforts. Everyone has a phone–computer, scrolling and clicking on the latest apps. Computer screens are used to scroll through computerized tomography (CT) scans of the human body, and modular health care record architecture allows the extension of product capabilities and interaction with other software programs. On hospital rounds, young physicians and students in a huddle are now armed with flat screens. They barely notice the patient and are quite unaware of their collective attention deficit disorder.

When compassionate readers of early fragments of these essays asked who the target audience of this communication would be, I replied that it would be all the Boomers so that they may perhaps better understand that they are all passengers on a large ship named the American health care industry (AHCI). Perhaps they can use some of the information provided here to influence their own fate. That is my wish.

The other potential audience that I hope may benefit from reading these pages is the next generations of American health care providers (a.k.a. doctors) now being trained to use the electronic media and to find their way through the fast-changing landscape of the AHCI. They deserve to know that medicine was not always like it is today and that there were times when we all used a simpler language and when doctors and nurses talked about patients, not about barriers that prevent access to care. AHCI has become a problem, and solutions are nowhere to be found.

During my four decades in medicine, I have witnessed vast progress and changes. Perhaps the greatest change has been the shift of emphasis from making an accurate diagnosis to effective treatment. We now take it for granted that the diseases are correctly diagnosed, and we expect a similar expediency and precision when it comes to the treatment plan. Here lies the challenge: There are too many diseases we cannot treat and many we cannot cure.

And then there is the other nasty reality: too many people the AHCI does not care for.

When in Doubt, See the Patient is a collection of essays. My hope is that, in the aggregate, they will provide a bit of history of what has happened in medicine and *to* medicine as our technology and diagnostic tools have improved. These travels through the landscape of American medicine have been my own travels, and autobiographical bits and pieces are jumping-off points. Long ago, a friend told me, "Only the personal is interesting—for the general stuff, consult the newspapers." And so I did, making sure that the quotes I lifted are as verbatim as possible. "Cutting and pasting" has become a favorite tool of authors writing on computer screens. This tool helped me to juxtapose and insert statements without taking them out of context. Another friend and early reader of these essays suggested uploading these chapters on the Internet as blog posts. I have so far resisted. In a book, all the pieces come together, and the dots are connected. My sole purpose in writing this short book is to provide the greater context so that we all can understand how badly broken the health care delivery system is.

This essay collection is also for my son, Marc, who works as a pulmonary and critical care physician in an intensive care unit (who is too much in love with his latest iPhone) and my wife, Angelika, a surgeon, who wanted me to not write these pages.[1]

---

1 Moore N. ,Askin E. The Health Care Handbook, Washington University in St. Louis, 2012.

Chapter 1

I Think I Can't Afford My Disease

Mattie was 77 years old and showed up in the Pulmonary Hypertension Clinic with her husband, who was clearly dedicated to her.

"So, why did you come to visit today?" I asked.

"My cardiologist says that I have pulmonary hypertension and I should see you," was her response.

"Why does he say that you have pulmonary hypertension? Did you bring any of your records?"

"He was supposed to send them to your office!"

I had nothing. This was her first visit. The referring cardiologist must have done an echocardiogram and other tests that were not available to me. Mattie's symptoms were "no energy" and "I am so short of breath just walking upstairs to our bedroom." In her past medical history, there were likely pulmonary blood clots. She had received a blood thinner for some years, maybe ten years earlier. With her husband looking on but saying little, I found out that her doctor—the cardiologist—had given her a prescription for Viagra, an erectile dysfunction drug for men that is also prescribed for the treatment of pulmonary hypertension in patients of either gender.

"You filled the prescription and started sildenafil?" I asked, using the other name for the drug, viagra.

"No, the pharmacist told me that my copay would be two thousand dollars a month! There is no way we can afford this. We are on Social Security, and I was a state employee. I have a small pension." She started crying.

Unfortunately, I was familiar with the situation, and I dreaded explaining next steps to her.

"Mattie, we may have to do a heart catheter study to find out how high the pressure in your lung circulation is. This is a procedure where a small tube is threaded, after puncture of your neck vein, through the large vessels into the right chamber of your heart and into the big pulmonary artery."

"Oh, I think I had this test," she said, perking up.

"All right, then your cardiologist should be so good and send me the results of this test."

Two weeks later, Mattie and her husband returned to the clinic for a second visit, this time armed with the heart catheterization report. Her husband had picked it up at the cardiologist's office. The report said that Mattie had severe pulmonary hypertension. The cardiologist had performed a test that showed that her pulmonary artery pressure could be brought down. She was a great candidate for treatment with the drug Viagra. I looked at the date of the catheter study; it indicated that the study had been done six months earlier. The patient had had symptoms for about a year and a diagnosis for six months—but no treatment. I wrote a prescription for sildenafil (Viagra) and told Mattie to go to her pharmacy.

The next day, the pharmacy called my office. Yes, they would give Mattie the pills, but a "prior authorization" from her insurance would be required. The friendly pharmacist gave me a toll-free phone number. I called the 866 number and, after trial and error, got to a human being. "The pharmacy instructed me to get prior authorization for Mattie...."

"What is the member's ID?" came the response.

I had the patient's ID and gave it to her.

"What is your DEA number?" I gave her my DEA number.

"What is the patient's diagnosis?"

"Severe pulmonary hypertension."

"What is your specialty?"

"I am a pulmonologist."

"Are we paying for this drug? We have not previously paid for this."

"Yes, this is a new prescription."

"We can try to expedite this. What is your fax number? I will fax you a form for an expedited prior authorization."

"Yes," I said, "I can fax you the form back in five minutes. How long is it going to take before Mattie can get her medicine?"

"It depends," the woman answered. "We have to check things out. By the way, do you see pulmonary hypertension patients on a regular basis?"

Mattie has Medicare, but this does not mean that she can afford this very expensive drug.

- When it comes to Medicaid, that is another matter altogether. Here is an excerpt from a recent assessment of the state of affairs:

Medicaid is the foundation of a vast expansion of publicly funded health insurance authorized by the Affordable Care Act (ACA). Medicaid is the country's single largest health insurer, with an average enrollment of fifty-five million. In recent years, as in previous state recessions, states have experienced large increases in Medicaid spending as more people become unemployed and enrolled in the program. To help close their budget benefits, some states are reducing payments to physicians, hospitals, and nursing homes. Some states have also reduced or restricted prescription drug benefits, raised or imposed new beneficiary copayments....

There is also no question that Medicaid patients with the most complex conditions could gain by enrolling in well-run managed-care plans that provide more integrated, readily accessible services than the uncoordinated fee-for-service model. But getting from here to there will be one of Medicaid's greatest challenges over the next decade, and physicians will have to play a leading role. Indeed, it's nothing less than a grand social experiment that bears closely watching by stakeholders of every stripe.[2]

Against this backdrop, Mattie, Medicare insured, has been eagerly watching and waiting. Is she a stakeholder? As far as I know, she is a patient who is not getting a medication that she needs. Increasingly, health care providers, a.k.a. doctors, are being put on the defensive, fighting endless battles with insurance companies and faceless gatekeepers on behalf of their patients.

"What kind of doctor are you?"

I guess I am a stakeholder.

Meanwhile, on a different floor of the hospital where I work, a well-insured (Platinum Plan) 35-year-old woman is being told that her tumor tissue can be subjected to a genetic analysis. Mutated genes and the

---

2 J.K. Iglehart, "Expanding Eligibility, Cutting Costs—A Medicaid Update," *New England Journal of Medicine* 366,no12(2012):105-107.

probability of response to chemotherapy, or targeted treatment, can be evaluated. Here is the context of genetic analysis of tumor tissues and the prospect of "personalized medicine."

> The fundamental idea behind personalized medicine is to couple established clinical-pathobiology indices with state-of-the-art molecular profiling to create diagnostic, prognostic, and therapeutic strategies precisely tailored to each patient's requirements—hence the term "precision medicine." Recent biotechnological advances have led to an explosion of disease-relevant molecular information, with the potential for greatly advancing patient care. However, progress brings new challenges, and the success of precision medicine will depend on establishing frameworks for regulating, compiling, and interpreting the influx of information.... In addition, we must make health care stakeholders aware that precision medicine is no longer just a blip on the horizon—and ensure that it lives up to its promise.[3]

I have contrasted Mattie's dilemma of not being able to afford her medicine with the options that the financially advantaged young cancer patient has. I don't know how many Matties there are in America or how we can decide who will be selected for personalized medicine. John Murray, one of the founding fathers of modern American pulmonary medicine, wrote in a recent editorial that "personalized medicine," the major clinical derivative of the hugely successful Human Genome Project—an approximately $3 billion monumental basic science research undertaking—is egregiously misnamed. The hype was launched when President Bill Clinton proclaimed that the achievement "would revolutionize the diagnosis, prevention, and treatment of most, if not all, human disease." John Murray is critical of the concept of personalized medicine as currently advertised, particularly when people get the impression that the concept has arrived "in the nick of time, so that doctors—at last—can start treating individual patients." He goes on:

---

3 R. Mirnezami, J. Nicholson, A. Darzi, "Preparing for Precision Medicine," *New England Journal of Medicinn e* 366,no 12(2012):489-91.

Haven't we been doing that? Certainly, I have always believed and taught students that doctors have practiced "personalized medicine" since 400 BC, thanks to Hippocrates, who actually did transform the practice of medicine by changing the treatment of sick people from magical potions and religious incantations to empirical remedies....[4]

I am with John Murray.

There are big tectonic faults that are constantly shifting and volcanoes ready to erupt any time now in this American health care landscape.

Although the use of the "r" word is taboo, rationing of health care uses will become unavoidable. Since American health care took the turn to industrialization, it has become very difficult to find the balance between making money and spending money. Practice guidelines and treatment algorithms are merely guidelines and subject to change. Medicine by committee consensus will be used to identify rationing rules, while the ethicists are debating how to establish loopholes and defend exceptions. When looking at printed diagnosis and treatment decision trees, I am always reminded of pinball machines. The ball is dropped at the top, bounces around, and escapes through a hole at the bottom. These algorithms are great didactic aids, expected to be used during hospital teaching rounds. I have difficulties applying these machines to the patients in my office. William Osler , the Canadian born patron saint of early twentieth century American medicine, said it best: "Were it not for the great variability among individuals, medicine might as well be science and not art."

A drug company recently sent out to physicians for free ("Download to your iPhone and iPad now!") a patient "risk score calculator" that displays, on one page that can be torn off, a "tearpad." It uses a scoring system that calculates "low risk" (predicted one-year survival: 95–100 percent) to "very high risk" (predicted one-year survival: less than 70 percent). The back page of this calculator reads: "It is our hope that widespread use of this risk score calculator will enable clinicians to individualize and optimize

---

4 J.F. Murray, "Personalized Medicine: Been There, Done That, Always Needs Work," *American Journal of Respiratory Critical Care* Medicine185,no 2(2012):1251-52.

therapeutic strategies." This is code for: "Doctor, you had better prescribe our drug!"

If there is the concept of "personalized medicine," is there a fear or a reality of "depersonalized" medicine? I am not percussing words. Does the choice of terms such as "industry," "clients," "care providers," "stakeholder," "care pool," and "health management association" tell us what is wrong with our profession?

Did you know that every year, hospitals generate twenty-eight pounds of medical waste per bed? What is this supposed to tell us? That we rely on single-use, throw-away, packaged supplies? We should talk about "medical waste" in an entirely different context.

In a recent paper, Jon Gabel and colleagues examined the health care "generosity" of several care plans to assess the out-of-pocket spending that is still required after health plans have kicked in. Here are some of their findings:

> "When beneficiaries use out-of-network providers, they incur much larger out-of-pocket expenses. The Affordable Care Act (ACA) sets up four tiers of health plans that people will be able to purchase with each tier defined by its actuarial value. The actuarial value measures the financial protection that the plan offers. If a plan has an actuarial value of 75 percent, the insurer pays three-fourths of the bills of that particular population—the members collectively pay one-fourth out of pocket in deductibles, copayments, and other cost sharing."[5]

In 2010, for families that incurred medical expenses that placed them in the top 1 percent of the group-plan-insured population, the plans paid 96 percent. For the bottom 50 percent, the plans paid only 64 percent of the charges.

For an average family, annual out-of-pocket expenses were $1,765 with group coverage, compared to $4,127 with individual coverage. Very sick

---

5 JR Gabel et al "More than half of individual health plans offer coverage that falls short of what can be sold through exchanges by 2014" Health Aff (Millwood) 6 (2012),1339-48.

patients—those in the top 1 percent, face out-of-pocket expenses of nearly $3,800 in a group insurance plan.

Then there was the case of Dr. Lukas Wartman.[6] As he was sending out letters applying for his residency training in 2003, he was diagnosed with acute lymphoblastic leukemia (ALL). Dr. Wartman received chemotherapy, had a remission, then experienced a recurrence that was treated with bone marrow transplantation (his brother's bone marrow). By the time the cancer recurred again, he had become an oncologist and was researching leukemia at the Washington University School of Medicine Hospital in St. Louis. His cancer researcher colleagues and friends decided to perform a full gene sequencing study of his cancer cells. This unique case does not end here and was recently reported in *The New York Times*. His cancer cell gene sequence analysis revealed that his leukemia cells highly expressed a cell growth factor gene. The good news was that a former small biotech company in south San Francisco, named Sugen, had developed a drug called Sutent (now marketed by Pfizer after the pharmaceutical giant bought the Sugen company). Sutent targets this particular growth factor receptor. The bad news was that Sutent costs $330 a day! Dr. Wartman's insurance company refused to pay for the drug, and Lukas Wartman lost two appeals. Pfizer's "compassionate drug use program" also turned him down. He then saved some money to buy a week's worth of the drug and, as his blood counts normalized, the doctors in the oncology division at Washington University chipped in and purchased a month's worth of Sutent.

Later in the year, Pfizer reconsidered and provided the drug for the doctor/patient/researcher.

What a vast and varied landscape this health care situation is. Every patient has a different disease and different prognosis, a different attitude, and different coping and healing mechanisms.

---

6 G. Kolata, "Genetic Gamble in Treatment of Leukemia, Glimpses of the Future." New York Times, July 7 2012.

Chapter 2

A Short Overview of the History of Health Insurance in America

The study of history is not a luxury.
Henry Sigerist

To understand where we are today, and why, it is helpful to review where we came from. It is of particular interest and importance to find out about the traditional and ongoing resistance of many stakeholders and legislators toward universal health care. Why this resistance in the United States and not in other countries? Why is America the only highly developed, indus-trialized country that does not offer universal health care? And why is it that politicians running for office continue to pronounce that the American health care system is the best in the world? "We are number one!"

> The absence of universal health insurance coverage is one of the great unsolved problems facing the nation at the onset of the twenty-first century. It has serious consequences for millions of uninsured Americans—their health, access to care, preventive care, and quality of care—as well as for those with inadequate health insurance. For example, those who are uninsured or underinsured are more likely not to have a regular doctor.... The Commonwealth Fund 1999 National Survey of Worker's Health Insurance found that 49 percent of the uninsured did not see a doctor when needed, did not fill a prescription due to cost. [7]

---

7 K. Davis, "Universal Coverage in the United States: Lessons from Experience of the 20th century," *Journal of Urban Health: Bulletin of the New York Academy of Medicine* (2001).

Donald Light, reflecting on US national health insurance reforms,[8] concludes that during the nineteenth century, charity hospitals were converted into fee-charging facilities and that "mainstream medicine...snuffed out national health insurance reform." In 1912, Theodore Roosevelt, in his bid for the presidency, endorsed health insurance modeled on workmen's compensation. In Germany in 1881, Otto von Bismarck introduced "sickness insurance" legislation, and in England in 1911, David Lloyd George sponsored the National Health Insurance Act. He did so stating the following:

"I think that now would be a very opportune moment for us in the homeland to carry through a measure that will relieve untold misery in myriads of homes, misery that is undeserved...in this country...thirty percent of the pauperism is attributable to sickness...."

The concepts that were behind the introduction of health insurance in both countries were similar.

"Social insurance, and this is in the widest sense of the word including even optional insurance, has to serve as a protection for the following cases of existence: when there is temporary impairment of the capacity for work, and with this of the earning power, whether this comes about through causes relating to the individual or through material conditions, namely:

- Through sickness
- Through accident
- Through child bearing and what follows
- Through poor conditions of the labor market."[9]

Amazingly, this approach to health care is driven by economics. Sick people are not productive; people who have lost their earning power are bad consumers—sickness causes pauperism. Is it possible that at the time of the

---

8 D.W. Light, "Historical and Comparative Reflections on the US National Health Insurance Reforms, *Social Science and Medicine* (2011).
9 M.M. David, "The American Approach to Health Insurance," The Milbank Memorial Fund Quarterly (1934).

establishment of the National Health Insurance Act in Britain (1911) and Theodore Roosevelt's endorsement of health insurance (1912), a fee-for-service machinery had already been so firmly entrenched that society was blind to the linkage of sickness and pauperism?

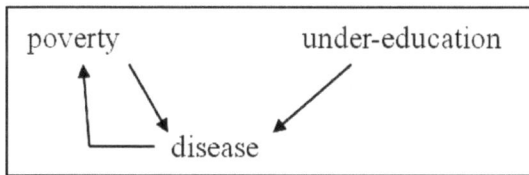

The United States has often lagged behind other nations in recognizing economic, social, and cultural rights, including the right to health.[10] Why?

We surely can understand the burden of disease as an economic burden. Why did American doctors—many trained in Germany early in the twentieth century—not import, together with their German anatomy textbooks, concepts of universal health insurance? Donald Light thinks the main reason is the "autonomous provider," who already in the 1970s formed group practices and converted practices into corporations that set up specialty clinics and, more recently, corporate imaging centers. Today, incorporated specialty group practices are the norm in urban America.

For quite some time, American doctors had well-developed business interests. An early example is Samuel S. Fitch, MD, who wrote a book about consumption[11] and sold a corset-like chest supporter.

10 M. McGill, "Human Rights from the Grassroots Up: Vermont's Campaign for Universal Health Care," Health Human Rights, 2012.

11 S.S. Fitch, Six Lectures on the Function of the Lungs (New York: J.H. Mackenzie, 1862).

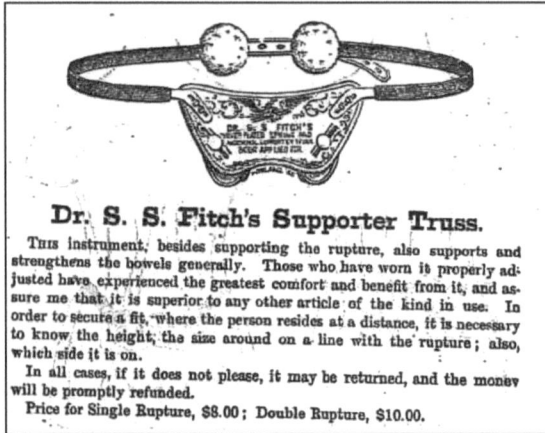

Dr. S. S. Fitch's Supporter Truss.

Tns instrument, besides supporting the rupture, also supports and strengthens the bowels generally. Those who have worn it properly adjusted have experienced the greatest comfort and benefit from it, and assure me that it is superior to any other article of the kind in use. In order to secure a fit, where the person resides at a distance, it is necessary to know the height; the size around on a line with the rupture; also, which side it is on.

In all cases, if it does not please, it may be returned, and the money will be promptly refunded.

Price for Single Rupture, $8.00 ; Double Rupture, $10.00.

He advertised his services and his group practice in 1861, during the early days of the Civil War:

"This is to certify that I have associated with me as partners in my practice L.E. King, MD, and I.E.B. Chambre, MD. I always prefer to have the opportunity of a personal examination of patients whenever it is possible and for this purpose desire that they should visit me at my office. But a personal examination is not indispensable. A statement of the symptoms and condition of the patient, with a full history of his disease, will enable me to prescribe and apply my treatment successfully without seeing the patient. My remedies can be sent with full directions to any part of the country."

Another prominent entrepreneurial physician was Alfred Coombs Barnes (1872–1915), who was born in Philadelphia and graduated from the medical school at the University of Philadelphia. He became a medical doctor at age twenty and a millionaire by the age of thirty-five. Together with Hermann Hille, Dr. Barnes developed a liquid silver nitrate antiseptic that he marketed under the name Argyrol®. The solution was used as a treatment for gonorrhea and to prevent gonorrheal blindness in newborns. Dr. Barnes started collecting art and, in 1922, established the Barnes Foundation, which, in a recently completed new building, houses his collection of sixty-nine Cezannes, sixty Matisses, and forty-four Picassos. I do not know of any charitable contributions that Dr. Barnes may have made as a gesture of gratitude to the medical sciences or to any health organization. The Barnes Hospital, later the Barnes–Jewish Hospital in St. Louis, was established by the bequest of a different Robert A. Barnes.

Reading about the history of American health insurance, one will sooner or later encounter Paul Starr's *The Social Transformation of American Medicine*. Here I make use of a later presentation of selected passages from the book titled *Precis of Paul Starr's The Social Transformation of American Medicine*. The book is now twenty years old, but it remains an astute analysis of the vexing health care problems of today, and it attempts to explain why universal health insurance was not established in the United States.

Understanding the prevailing forces and barriers that have been working against the greater good is now more important than it was in 1982. Here we are not examining the cost of doing nothing, but we follow Paul Starr's line of reasoning, which starts with the statement that medicine is a world of power and authority and a fraternity of professionals who continue to fight for their autonomy.

Starr explains the following:

"Power originates in dependence, and the power of the (medical profession) primarily originates in dependence upon the knowledge and competence of the profession. Unlike the law and the clergy, the medical profession enjoys bonds with modern science, and the medical practitioners come into intimate contact with people at critical transitional moments of their existence: birth and death. Physicians offer personal relationships and authoritative counsel".[12]

Lawyers have always had great difficulties in accepting this special and elevated position of the medical profession. After all, sometimes they make life-and-death decisions, too, which now, ironically, can be overruled by unassailable DNA evidence.

Starr is interested in the roots of the authority of the medical profession. Doctors claim authority as members of a community endowed with

---

12 P. Starr, The Social Transformation of American Medicine (New York: Basic, 1982).

special knowledge and validated standards. The knowledge is applied in accordance with critically evaluated guidelines, which are directed toward improving health and reducing pain and suffering. This service orientation can clash with the profit orientation..

Authority can be converted into high income if the market (the health care industry) does not take over the control of the institutions that govern medical practice, financing, and health care policy. The emergence of professional authority was, at the outset, not automatically tied to the conversion of the healing arts into a commercial enterprise. "Medicine...has historically distinguished itself from business and trade by claiming to be above the market and pure commercialism.(P. Starr)"

Ronald Reagan, the "great communicator," assured the American people that there was nothing special about the medical profession—the health care industry was an industry like any other industry. "Ever since the market has eroded the authority of the health care profession—and most ironically the highly valued autonomy meant that one could practice medicine where one wanted to practice, and—without many restrictions and regulations "(P. Starr). Autonomy in 2013 is pretty much gone.

I am still stunned when I read Paul Starr's 1982 conclusion today: "The doctors escaped becoming victims of capitalism and became small capitalists instead."

The equation increasingly has become as follows:
Knowledge + authority = market power + profit
Rather than:
Knowledge + authority = reduction of pain + suffering

Traditionally, doctors have been opposed to corporate structures and influences because they wanted autonomy but also because they did not want to share profits with a third party. That has changed. We now have the Hospital Association of America.

Under the headline "Capitalism and the Doctors," Paul Starr writes, "The American Medical Association (AMA) stated in a section of its code of ethics adopted in 1934 that it was 'unprofessional for a physician to permit a "direct profit" to be made from his work.

The making of a profit from medical work is beneath the dignity of the professional practice, is unfair competition with the profession at large, is harmful alike to the profession of medicine and the welfare of the people, and is against public policy. Not that the AMA believed it was wrong for doctors to make profit from their work. Nor did it reprimand the physician owners of medical groups for making a profit off the work of other doctors. The AMA opposed anyone else, such as an *investor* (the italics are mine) making a return from physicians' labor. The AMA was saying, in short, that there must be no capital formation in medical care (other than what doctors accumulated), that the full return on physicians' labor had to go to physicians, and consequently, by implication that if medicine required any capital that doctors could themselves not provide, it would have to be contributed *gratis* by the community. Physicians did not want to be subjected to the kind of hierarchical controls that typically prevail in industrial capitalism.

Since 1934, corporate America has successfully invaded the medical profession, and the government is in control of the pay line. The once-unique personal relationship between patient and doctor has changed because the industry treats doctors as producers, hospitals as production sites, and patients as consumers"(P.Starr).

Baby Boomers, be aware: You are not really being diagnosed with and treated for an illness—you are consumers of health care.

Table 1 shows, in chronological order, the major initiatives and, so far, failed attempts to move American health care to universal coverage.

Table 1. National health insurance proposals

Theodore Roosevelt	1912
Social Security Act	1935
Harry Truman: Adding universal health insurance to Social Security	1945
Dwight D. Eisenhower: Market reforms	1954
Lyndon B. Johnson: Medicare and Medicaid Act	1965
Richard Nixon: Comprehensive Health Insurance Plan	1971
Jimmy Carter:National Health Plan	1979
Pepper Commission chaired by Senator Jay Rockefeller	1990

George H. BushVouchers	1992
Bill ClintonClinton Health Security	1994
State Children Health Insurance Plan	1997
Barack Obama: Affordable Care Act(ACA)	2012

How to go from here is likely going to be decided by the people who voted to re-elect the president of the United States in 2012. "The outcome of the 2012 election will have far-reaching ramifications for the future of US health care. Health care and Medicare ranked second after "economy and jobs" among the most important issues for voters in the 2012 presidential election."[13]

---

13 R.J. Blendon, et al. "Understanding Health Care in the 2012 Election," New England Journal of Medicine 367, no. 17 (2012) 1658-61.

Chapter 3

Global Payments and Opportunity in Austerity

My father-in-law practiced as a general surgeon in a small town on the border between Ohio and Kentucky. Every ten years or so, the Ohio River flooded the low-lying areas of Sioto County. For a few days, the road would become impassable until the water retreated, leaving the mud behind and humidity, which made all creation dripping wet. My father-in-law delivered all of the babies in Sioto County for more than twenty years, and as they grew up, they became big and rotund people and his patients.

As was later explained to me, he emigrated with his wife and three girls from postwar Germany in 1949, which was unusual during those times. My wife's uncle had worked with Wernher von Braun and would later join the team that launched the Apollo Space Program and built the space shuttle and space station. I remember Uncle Hans and his excitement about space as a new frontier as he explained how we could manufacture new proteins and crystals in zero gravity. Postwar Germany was still in ruins in 1949 and America the Promised Land, where people were generous and had open minds. Rural Ohio needed doctors, and they wanted my wife's dad to come and practice medicine. They could not have made a better choice.

After high school in Ohio, my future wife attended Stuart Hall, the Institute for Young Women founded by Jeb Stuart's widow, Mary, after the Civil War. Staunton in Virginia was a day's travel over winding mountain roads from Sioto County, and Stuart Hall was preparatory, but not for medical school. In the sixties, women had practically no chance to get admitted to medical school. As the Dean of Ohio State Medical School would explain to me while doing a four-month externship a few years later, "The girls get married and then they have babies.... We just can't afford to train them for that." A typical American medical school class in the sixties consisted of one hundred students, with only four or five of them women. My future wife was shipped to Grandma, who resided in the south of Germany, and she enrolled in the medical school of the ancient University of Würzburg, the place where Wilhelm Roentgen had discovered x-rays. That's where I met my wife. Back in Ohio, during the turbulent summer of 1968, while enrolled in an externship at Ohio State Medical School in Columbus, I visited my in-laws and got a first impression of rural, private-practice medicine. My father-in-law had a legendary Saturday clinic for the people who could not take time off from work during the week. He had a small office building where Thelma, the nurse resided, dressed in a sparkling white uniform, complete with a starched hat. She knew everybody and everything. My father-in-law performed surgery in two of the Portsmouth hospitals, but on Saturdays he was in the office from eight in the morning until two or two-thirty to see thirty or forty patients; he would examine them, and the exam was spiced with a joke or two. He would order tests, prescribe medicine, and hand out medication samples. Yes, doctors had samples to give out in those days, an accepted way to help poor people. "You don't have your paycheck yet? Then take this sample," he would say.

One Saturday, I picked my father-in-law up as he was about to finish his clinic. He asked Thelma to show me the day's revenue. "Thelma, can you show my son-in-law what we got paid today?" Thelma handed me a stack of checks about half an inch thick. She would later log them in the day's ledger, but for then, there was the stack, and each check was made out for ten, twenty, or twenty-five dollars. That was it. No bill. Thelma knew what to charge, and Mrs. Kitts and Mr. Peebles wrote a check—or if they could not write the check that Saturday, they came back a week later with a blueberry pie in a pan, and the check was sitting on top of it.

Most people had work, regular pay, and some kind of health insurance. For the Saturday morning clinic visit, they paid out of pocket. They could, and they wanted to.

The term "health care system" had not been invented then. There were simply doctors, nurses, and hospitals. Life was simple. Doctors made house calls; the pharmacist knew the patient and the doctor. There were no health care access problems, no payment defaults, and no claims adjustors.

Of course, this is all very distant and hard to believe. I reminisce about these good old days because our medical profession has forgotten this part, this uncomplicated, fascinatingly unregulated style of practicing medicine.

The medical students of the class of 2014 can't imagine what it was like.

Now we are dealing with money traps in US healthcare, issues of medical claims and billing, armies of administering inspectors and accountants in business attire, electronic medical recordkeeping, and three-day, high-intensity training courses that prepare lawyers for the business of suing doctors and hospitals in the skilled reading of these electronic records: The cardiologist wrote on Monday...but the oncologist stated on Wednesday.... Wait a minute. What is going on here is malpractice!

Medicaid claims have gone before the Supreme Court, and a recent report from the Organization for Economic Cooperation and Development (OECD), a thirty-four-member group that includes the most advanced industrial nations, concluded that healthcare spending in the United States is high partly because the prices charged by American doctors and hospitals are higher than anywhere else. An appendectomy costs four times more in the United States than in Germany, and an MRI (magnetic resonance imaging) study costs three times as much here as in Canada. Germany, Italy, and Japan have a greater percentage of elderly citizens than the United States, but spending is much less per capita on health care. The United States spends $8,000 per person annually on health care, about 50 percent more than Switzerland spends. Hospital stays are very costly, at $18,000 per discharge, compared to less than $10,000 in France or Germany.

In departmental meetings, the department's annual income or revenue is reported and discussed. Physicians are being paid according to revenue-generating units. Sitting in those meetings, I have noticed that the charts and graphs show an average increase in departmental revenues of about 10 percent each year; over a period of five years this amounts to a revenue increase of greater than 50 percent.

The captains of the health care providers, the hospital CEOs, know their marching orders. Do not forget Reagan's words: "The American health care industry is an industry like any other industry." The health care industry markets and advertises services, not different from the travel or financial industries or the pharma industry. What hospital executive worth his or her salt will not think about how to maximize profit?

That's where *primum nil nocere* (first do no harm) clashes with primum profit..

The "industry of medical care" concept is remarkable for its internal consistency, and the industry does not deliver what it promises to deliver. For example, the magnitude of pain in the United States is astounding. More than 116 million Americans have pain that persists for weeks or years. The total financial costs of this epidemic are $560 billion to $635 billion per year. According to a report of an Institute of Medicine Committee titled "Relieving Pain in America," relieving acute and chronic pain is a significant and overlooked problem in the United States:

> Major impediments to the relief (of pain) include patients' limited access to clinicians who are knowledgeable about acute and chronic pain—owing in part to the prevalence of outmoded or unscientific knowledge of attitudes about pain.... More than 65 percent of nursing home residents report having inadequately treated pain. Decisions about medical care are also influenced by insurance coverage that may be preferential for injections, infusions, procedures, and surgery over physical therapy, rehabilitation, and more comprehensive approaches to pain control.[13]

And this is where it really hurts; the report goes on:

> A major challenge is the limited education that US medical students and physicians receive about pain. A survey of 117 medical schools showed that some included in their curricula only a few educational sessions on pain. The deficiency carries over to professional education: Half of primary care physicians report feeling

---

14 P.A. Pizzo and N.M. Clark, "Alleviating Suffering 101—Pain Relief in the United States," *New England Journal of Medicine* 366, no. 3 (2012) 197-99.

only "somewhat prepared" to counsel patients about pain, and 27 percent feel "somewhat unprepared" or "very unprepared."[14]

While there is not enough talk about pain and suffering, many physicians receive detailed instructions on how to structure their interactions with patients and their physical exam—"for billing purposes." The medical history can be "problem-focused," "extended," or "comprehensive." The number of organ systems reviewed and examined can vary from eight to twelve body areas, such as head, neck, abdomen, and each extremity. The number of diagnoses matters, as does the number of management issues. It matters how many medications the patient takes and whether drug allergies, side effects of drugs, and drug interactions have been discussed. The correlation—if any—between symptoms and findings and the other lab and imaging data needs to be documented in great detail.

I don't remember when it was exactly, but sometime after 2000, flat screens multiplied like rabbits and began to populate American hospitals. Flat screens and keyboards are now everywhere—outside of patients' rooms, in the nurses' stations, in the doctors' offices, and in the patients' rooms. Receptionists in the clinics hardly look at the patient; they enter data and print out copies of Social Security cards. Once upon a time, a nurse was someone who talked with patients, fed patients, and helped them into the chair. Now a nurse updates the medical record, and the computer screen wedges itself between the nurse and the patient.

"Hi, Tennessee. Let me get your story up on my computer," I say as I try to reconcile the patient sitting on my left with the data on the screen in front of me. I am confused by the pop-up windows that tell me about things that I don't want to know or to do. Large health care investments have been made in hardware and software and in seminars on health policy. In recent publications, you can read the following techno-statement:

A health care system responsible for meeting requirements could conceivably partner in such an endeavor with a public health

15 N.W Skine. And D.A Chokshi. "Opportunity in Austerity-A Common Agenda for Medicine and Public Health." *New England Journal of Medicine* 366, no. 5 (2012): 395-97.

institution that is already engaged in activities but that might lack the funds necessary to fully assess and address identified needs. A partnership built on the financial and technological resources of hospitals and the broader perspective and population management expertise of the public health sector could serve as a blueprint for future community collaborations on the other common goals, such as reduction of hospital admissions.[15]

The hospital close to the Atlantic coast I am working in at the time of this writing serves a community that is 52 percent African American. Greater than 90 percent of the one thousand or so hospital beds are always filled. The emergency room is the place of first—and for many patients the *only*—encounter with health care, and overflowing. This ER has a control and command center where each patient is tracked on giant flat screens. Numbers and

messages pop up and disappear, constantly monitored by ER doctors. Patients are admitted to the hospital as a bed becomes available after they had been routed to the CT scanner. Patients who have been admitted will have most of their tests done within forty-eight hours after admission. The reimbursements to the hospital decline thereafter.

Hospitals, very much like Home Depot or Walmart, can advertise—and they do. Consider this hospital's promotional language:

"The hospital has completed a $100 million expansion and has increased its campus size by 50 percent, introducing new services and expanded offerings while providing clients with easy access to the most visited areas. The expansion has doubled the square footage of the emergency room, enabling the ER team to serve two thousand more patients; the expansion has allowed for the opening of the Cancer Specialty Clinic, where the multidisciplinary clinics have expanded from two disease states to five (breast, prostate, lung, colorectal, and hepatobiliary.) Increased office space has brought an additional twenty-plus physicians to practice on the campus..."[16].

16 Richmond, VA, regional hospital advertisement, 2012.
17 Invitation to "Dealmaking Summit" by unsolicited e-mail.

An invitation to attend the Annual Healthcare Dealmaking Summit reads as follows:

"Industry players gather to analyze health care and the impacts of public policy for patient flow in 2013. The Healthcare Dealmaking Summit brings together buyers, sellers, financiers, middlemen, and other essential players.... Record levels of deal-making activity have been a creative response to the ongoing evolution of the American health care sector."[17]

The share of the workforce employed in the health care industry, relative to the total non-farming civilian workforce, has increased between 1975 and 2010 from 0.05 percent to 0.1 percent—it has doubled. And the cost per year to generate a one-year increase in life expectancy also doubled during the same period, from $125,000 to more than $250,00[18]. In contrast to, let's say, the car industry, in which fewer and fewer workers produce greater numbers of cars, in the health care industry more and more health care providers are generating more health care costs. The salaries for the growing armies of health care workers have to be paid by someone. Further increasing the numbers of employees in this industry flies in the face of the concept of better health care for fewer dollars.

---

18 K. Baicker and A. Chandra," The Health Care Jobs Fallacy," New England Journal of Medicine 366, no. 26 (2012): 2433-35.

Chapter 4

Bundled Care

As I was taking my lunch in the postmodern cafeteria of the Free University Medical Center in Amsterdam, the Netherlands—a pulmonary hypertension symposiumin 2012 had brought me there—the American nation, deeply divided over stem cells, global warming, and creationism, found itself in the Supreme Court arguing the constitutionality of the Affordable Care Act (ACA). With *The New York Times* piece on the Supreme Court's proceedings displayed on my computer, I looked at the PhotoShopped spoof version of Rembrandt's *Anatomy of Doctor Tulp* (the original is displayed in the Maurits Museum in Den Haag), which shows the good doctor Tulp lifting the claw of a red lobster instead of the dissected hand shown in the original.

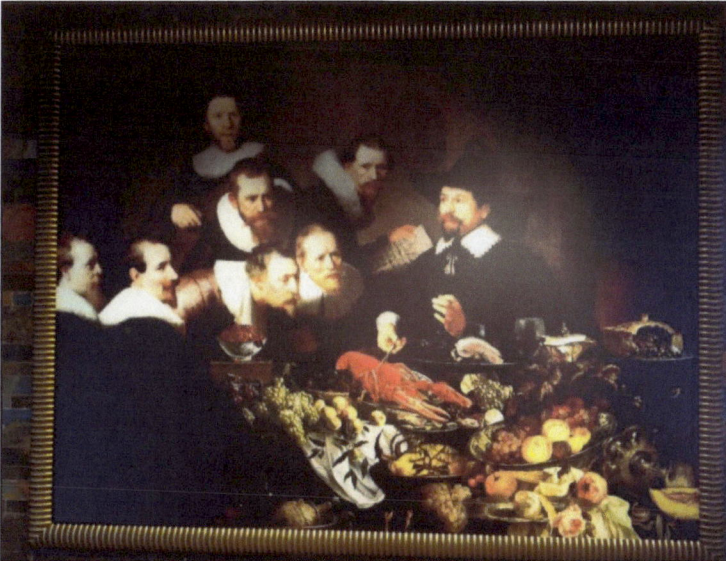

We do not make health care jokes in the United States. "Robama scare" was one of the favorite stump speech topics on the presidential election topics list, and Romney/Obama health care plans—past and future—were dissected on the Sunday-morning TV talk shows.

Twenty-six US states challenged the health care law. The defense stated that there is "a profound connection between health care and liberty," while the opponents answered that "it is a very funny conception of liberty that forces somebody to purchase an insurance policy whether they want it or not."[19]

Yet it is not funny that in most of the US states, car insurance is mandatory—it is the law. Justice Anthony Kennedy said, "By denying any one government complete jurisdiction over all the concerns of public life, federalism protects the liberty of the individual from arbitrary power."[17] The protection of the individual from arbitrary power should be examined in the context of the limited access of many individuals to health care and compared with the approach that the Dutch Government has taken to provide universal health care, as we will see later.

On one of the days I was there, Amsterdam was ready for spring; the Vondel Park was filled with people who had taken this Friday off to take their girlfriends and new babies to a picnic in the park. Before lunch in the cafeteria, I had listened in on a discussion regarding a patient with lung cancer. His cancer was advanced and had eroded into the esophagus, and stent placement for the trachea and esophagus were contemplated—and hospice, which I will address later.

In the United States, an enormous amount of money is spent on care during the last months of life, and the politicization of end-of-life debates,[20] the specter of "death panels," and stakeholder positions in a religion-based culture continue to distort the real situation of the sick and elderly. "The philosophy behind much current policy—including ACA—is that aggregating fee-for-service reimbursement into payments for broader bundles of care will lead to greater efficiency in the provision of care and thus lower costs.[21]

---

19 A. Liptake, The New York Times, In Health Case, Appeals to a Justice's Idea of Liberty, March 30, 2012.

20 S. Jacoby, The New York Times, "Taking Responsibility for Death," March 30, 2012.

21 D.M. Cutler and K. Gosh, "The Potential for Cost Saving through Bundled Episode Payments," New England Journal of Medicine (March 22, 2012).

I wonder: Is it "bungling" or "bundling"?

While the quest to manage US health care costs has inspired the health care industry to contemplate both episode-bundled payments and patient-based bundled payments to the providers, the US Supreme Court examines the ACA for "severability" of programs. Authors said the following in a *New England Journal of Medicine* article:

- "With 78 million Baby Boomers becoming eligible for Medicare over the next eighteen years, eventually doubling the number of beneficiaries, increased spending due to population aging, greater longevity is making the change to raise Medicare's eligibility from sixty-five to sixty-seven compelling.[21]

On the health care supply side, tight credit markets and shrinking endowments led to cancellation of capital projects."[21]

Both of these statements focus on the industry and beneficiaries. Cost and payment issues are examined, and profit margins by hospitals are being discussed in the context of the Tax Equity and Fiscal Responsibility Act of 1982, which apparently "left the hospitals with no upside,"[21] causing them to reduce the costs per admission by shortening the lengths of stay—which, in turn, has unfortunately led to a large increase in hospital readmission rates.

What we are looking at here is a mess—perhaps a bundled mess. Readmissions need to be avoided—as anyone knows, one can get sick in hospitals.

Can we ever come to grips with the health care problem in the United States? One is reminded of the image titled *Relativity* from the Dutch woodcut and lithography print artist M.C. Escher, which shows the optical illusion of faceless people endlessly climbing staircases without ever gaining elevation.

So, through "bundling" and keeping beneficiaries out of the hospitals, we will arrive at better health care? I think not!

Perhaps the most off-putting side of this multifaceted problem is the language that has evolved, the health-techno speak, the layers on layers of commentaries, and the bellicose posturing of the representatives of both political parties, with no practical solution in mind. Statements like "the American health care system is the best in the world" are untrue and unhelpful.

If that statement were true, then why are idealistic health care providers, dentists, eye doctors, nurses, and other specialists traveling to the boonies to pull teeth, fit eyeglasses, and check diabetes medicines—for free? And why are several hundred patients camping out and standing in line for such services—as recently was the case in West Virginia?

A recent article analyzes the goals of national value-based purchasing programs[22] and emphasizes six "domains of measurements," shown below, which can be affected only if the caregivers are properly incentivized—through a Quality Incentive Program (QIP), whose elements include the following:

- Safety
- Patient and caregiver-centered experience and outcomes
- Care coordination
- Clinical care
- Population or community health
- Efficiency and cost reduction

If the American health care system is the best in the world, then why is it so desperately seeking improvement, and why does it need a QIP?

Meanwhile, American doctors are soldiering on—mostly in silence, but burning out! I can't help it. I am going to rap:

A bundled care is a mess
Because it is less
Than optimal care
And more of a scare
For those who do not prepare
For their last months and the fare.

---

22 J.M. Van Lare and P.H. Conway, "Value-Based Purchasing—National Programs Move from Volume to Value," New England Journal of Medicine 367, no. 21 (2012) 2060.

Chapter 5

The Girl Who Died Twice

My decision to defect, to leave the University Hospital in Hamburg–Eppendorf, matured slowly. My surgeon father-in-law arranged for an externship in medicine—four months at Ohio State Medical School in Columbus. This experience forever changed my concepts of learning and teaching medicine. Being taught by professors in groups of four or five students about diseases, treatments, and side effects of drugs; by older residents about electrolyte disorders and cardiac arrhythmias; and by chief residents who visited the on-call team at midnight to prepare them for the questions they would get during the next day's morning report were experiences I could not forget. At Hamburg, there was little formal teaching for the medical residents. Instead of spoon feeding, there was mostly self-study. You figured it out yourself or you did not.

After several years of residency in internal medicine, I had flashbacks. Vivid images of training sessions in Columbus flooded my memory, and I started to keep a record of the days when I had been taught or had learned anything new. After six months of this practice, I looked at my desktop calendar and counted the "learned something new" days. My Chief of Medicine, whom I worshipped, was about to retire; one of the pulmonary medicine attending physicians had bluntly told me, "If you really want to do pulmonary research, you have to leave Germany." My surgeon wife, with her US passport, was agreeable to close our apartment in Eppendorf and apply for a research fellowship. I was ready. The Max Kade Foundation provided a stipend salary for one year. A year earlier, I had visited the Cardiovascular Pulmonary Laboratory at the University of Colorado in Denver, and Bob Grover, the director, had recommended that I apply to the foundation. So I did.

Nine months into my fellowship in Denver, I received a letter from Hamburg–Eppendorf, from the associate chief of medicine, which said in so many words, "Now that your time in the United States comes to an end, I want to notify you that you *will* return to your former position in the University Hospital, and you *will* start your duties running the general medicine admissions unit." It contained thirty beds, and all of the non-intensive-care patients were initially worked up on this ward. Not only had I served on this ward before for six months—I had done the rotation twice. That was clearly meant to be punishment for the care-free research year in America, the care-free year in the lab without patient care.

I told my wife that I would not do the admissions unit a third time. A week later, I wrote back to Hamburg that I would not return. I got a green card and sat for several written exams. The Internal Medicine Training Program director, Bob Schrier, a famous nephrologist, told me that I would get credit for my years of training in Hamburg, but I needed to do six months of medical internship without pay. There we were in Denver, my wife and I and our two children. We jumped, naively confident in our abilities. Somehow we would make it.

What the qualifying internship meant was that I admitted patients every third day, which meant that I started the call day at eight in the morning, admitted patients alternating with the second on-call team throughout the day and the night, while the next on-call team came on at eight the next morning. We residents stayed on, visited all of the team's patients, and worked up the newly admitted patients. We were interrupted only by the morning report and the noon conference. This pattern repeated itself every third day. The high point was breakfast at six in the morning after the call night was almost over. Was I tired? Yes. Was there time for the family? For socializing? Not really. We planned dinner parties with friends according to the call schedule—one month ahead of time.

My internship had been designed without any easy sub-specialty rotations giving me a break; if a patient on my service "crashed," I followed the patient into the intensive care unit, where he or she was not handed off to a special ICU team. "My patient—all the time" was the code of honor. Residents were extremely proud to manage their patients well, and we were protective of our patients. Toward the end of the third training year, usually during the months of May and June, residents reduced the subspecialty consultant doctors' input, almost insultingly telling the consult service attending physician: "You may see this patient for your own interest—but we don't ask for a consult!"

Of course, all of this was a long time ago, and all of it has changed dramatically. Residents are ordered to leave the hospital after call night at one in the afternoon, and no longer do chief residents "pimp" the on-call interns at midnight. The rules and regulations for medical training were made by the Council of Medical Education, established in 1904. Since 1981, the training oversight remains in the hands of the Accreditation Council for Graduate Medical Education (ACGME).

Things have changed, and it was the case of Libby Zion [23] that had the great impact on how residents were to train in US hospitals. In March 1984, Libby Zion died from serotonin syndrome in a New York City Hospital. Libby Zion was a freshman at Bennington College. She had been admitted to the hospital via the emergency department with fever, agitation, and jerking motions of her body. She had had a history of depression and had been treated with the monoamine oxidase inhibitor phenelzine (Nardil). Libby died from a drug-induced disease, and her death was investigated. A grand jury trial report was widely publicized. Libby's father wrote in an op-ed piece in *The New York Times*: "You don't need kindergartens to know that a resident working a thirty-six-hour shift is in no condition to make any kind of judgment call—forget about life and death." The image of overworked, undersupervised residents stuck. In 1989, New York State adopted the Bell Commission's recommendations that residents could not work more than eighty hours a week or more than twenty-four consecutive hours and that senior physicians needed to be physically present in the hospital at all times. In 2003, ACGME made reduced work hours mandatory for the accreditation of residency training programs across the United States. In 1991, the Appeal Court of the State of New York cleared the records of the two residents taking care of Libby Zion that fateful night, finding that they had not provided inadequate care to Libby Zion. How the Appeal Court came to this conclusion remains unclear. In 2010, the Institute of Medicine released

---

23 Natalie S. Robins, The Girl Who Died Twice. Dell, 1996.

a report recommending even stricter work-hour reductions and concluding that supervision of young physicians remained inadequate.[24,25].

Thinking back, I remember dozing off after a night on call during morning report. But I never handed off any of my patients during the time of my qualifying internship; they were very much my patients.

There is, of course, no turning back. The maturation process of physicians in training has been slowed down, and the time it takes for physicians to reach independent judgment and decision making has been extended. The training wheels come off later and later, and some physicians are uncomfortable with decision making; they look for a committee to help them. "Float" systems and mandatory leave after call have undoubtedly fragmented care, and taking responsibility is frequently replaced with a reflex dependence on a battery of consultants. Shift-working doctors often miss the evolution of a disease process, and, upon return for their next shift, find out that their patient no longer is their patient. The patient is now in the ICU or on the operating table.

"What happened?" they ask.

Hurried handoffs of patients at shift change now have replaced checkout rounds where the chief resident drills the incoming team: "The patient is sort of stable now—what will you do when X, Y, or Z happens? You should be prepared for this and that...."

In my opinion, the pendulum has swung too far from autonomy to supervision. Medical students are mostly pure observers, and a long apprenticeship is now associated with loss of ownership. This void is now filled with residents' "lifestyle" decisions made easier by schedules consisting of two weeks on and two weeks off.

Sidney Zion, Libby's father, has changed medical training in the United States forever. Yet July 1, the "independence day" for residents—the day on which they have fulfilled their training requirements—is increasingly approached with palpitations and tremors.

---

24 B.L. Lerner, "A Case that Shook Medicine," The Washington Post, November 28, 2006.

25 B.L. Lerner, "A Life-Changing Case for Doctors in Training," The New York Times, August 14, 2011.

But before "independence day," there are the Internal Medicine Program expectations regarding the "daily work" on in-patient services. These expectations read as follows:

- Interns are "in" between 5:30 and 6:00 a.m. They get the sign-out from the night floats. The handoff must be face to face.
- Pre-rounds include examination and interim (since hand-off) patient history.
- Work rounds start daily at 7:00 a.m.
- Residents and interns should see "sick or emergent" patients together.
- Consult requests should be called between 7:30 and 8:00 a.m.

Documentation:

- Should focus on assessment and plan—do not cut and paste from day before. Notes must be completed by 1:00 p.m. each day.
- Attending rounds must finish by 10:30 a.m. to start morning report at 11:00 a.m.
- Checkout rounds with attending—mandatory—4:00–6:00 p.m.
- One team member must remain in the hospital until sign-out to night team member at 7:00 p.m.—must occur in person.
- All house staff must attend morning report, Grand Rounds, and the didactic lectures, 3:00–6:00 p.m. on Tuesdays...

This list of expectations may sound or look reasonable to some, but what is missing is the heart of the matter. What is missing is a statement like this: "We expect that the residents know everything about their patients, that they—and not someone else—take responsibility for the care of their patients." Presumably, these expectations are passed on with the handoff and the fragmentation of care.[26]

---

26 VCU, Department of Internal Medicine, memorandum, 2012.

Chapter 6

Only the Hypothesis Enables You to See what Can Be Seen

The Cardiovascular Pulmonary research laboratory (CVP lab) in Denver was the place to do research in the areas of lung circulation and pulmonary hypertension. After several years of monitoring the journals and publications in this field, I could not fail to notice that the overwhelming number of new papers and ideas about pulmonary hypertension emanated from the Rocky Mountains. At the end of the Second World War, Ulf von Euler, together with Gustav Liljestrand, discovered that the pressure in the lung vessels increased when animals breathed a gas mixture that was low in oxygen. Originally called the v. Euler–Liljestrand "reflex," it was soon discovered that this response was no reflex at all because the increase in the lung vascular pressure occurred by contraction of the vessels also when all the nerves were severed and the lung was studied *ex vivo*—out of the body, isolated, and perfused with a physiologic salt solution.

During my training in the University Hospital in Hamburg, I discovered pulmonary hypertension and lung circulation. One night, on call for the internal medicine service, my pager gave alarm. I called the hospital telephone center and was directed to see a patient on the sixth floor. The hallways were all dark, and the wards were dark and quiet except for the nurses' station, where I was greeted by the night nurse. As I arrived on the floor two hours past midnight, the nurse told me that the patient had just died and that I needed to "pronounce her." The patient's room was dark except for a table lamp on the nightstand. There lay a young woman, her eyes closed, motionless. I pulled my stethoscope out of my white coat and listened to the nonexistent heart sounds, watched by the nurse. "When did she die?" I asked her.

"A few minutes ago," she said.

There was nothing to do. I went to the nurses' station and started to read the chart that the nurse had put on the table for me. The woman was twenty-nine years old and had been given the diagnosis of "primary pulmonary hypertension." I knew nothing about it but realized it was an ailment one could die from. A heart catheter study had been performed months earlier and revealed that the pressure in the lung circulation was extremely high, and shortly thereafter the young woman had developed signs and symptoms of heart failure. Reading from the last entries in the chart backward to the beginning, I learned that the young woman had had a baby and had gained some weight during her pregnancy. She wanted to lose weight and fit into her bikini and, upon request, had received a weight-loss medication with the name Menocil, which she had taken for six months. Soon after, it was discovered that this anorexigen (appetite suppressant) caused pulmonary hypertension. The drug was taken off the market in the three countries where it had been sold: Switzerland, Austria, and Germany. It turned out that the drug was, for some people, like a ticking time bomb. Pulmonary hypertension could even develop several years after the last pill had been taken. Within one year after the drug was approved cardiologists in the three countries observed a dramatic increase in primary pulmonary hypertension, and the common denominator, the weight-loss pill Menocil, was quickly identified as the cause of the disease.

It took me about half an hour to read through the chart and to understand that the young woman had succumbed to a drug-induced disease that was fatal. At the time of this woman's death, the drug had been off the market for almost three years. A silent killer.

The next day, post-call, I was determined to learn more about this disease. I knocked at the office door of one of the cardiologist attendings, and after I told him that I had had to pronounce a young woman with primary pulmonary hypertension dead the previous night, I asked him, "Who does take care of these patients? And what research is going on?"

He briefly looked up from the article he was editing and said, "You know, these patients have a lung vessel disorder—the pulmonologists take care of them."

So I went to see one of our pulmonologist attendings, and after telling him about my nocturnal experience, he said, "You know, these patients all die from right-sided heart failure. These patients belong to the cardiologists." I also learned that there was no early diagnosis and no treatment; the patients simply died. The year was 1974.

Still in Hamburg, I joined a small group of young physicians who shared an interest in lung diseases. One of the pulmonary attendings encouraged me to do research in the area of lung vascular diseases.

On the large campus of the Hamburg University hospital studded with red brick pavilions, which had been built around 1900, there was a small animal facility that had a mid-size hypoxia chamber—a steel box with an attached vacuum pump, generating a low-oxygen-pressure environment to simulate altitude exposure. The animals would be exposed to conditions simulating 15,000 or 17,000 feet above sea level, and over a period of three to four weeks, they would develop pulmonary hypertension due to chronic hypoxia. We had a model of pulmonary hypertension, the same model used by the pioneering and beautiful pathologist Lynn Reid in London, who had described that the lung vessels would get a thick muscle layer after the animals were in the hypoxia chamber. But, as I was trying to relate the animal model to the disease that had killed the young woman, I had no hypothesis.

Three years later, now working in the CVP lab in Denver, as a post-doctoral fellow, one of my mentors in this boot camp for aspiring researchers, Jack Reeves, seized on this. As soon as I got to the lab, I learned from a medical student how to isolate and perfuse the lungs of a rat, fascinated as I was with the hypoxic pressor response of the isolated lung. There were hundreds, perhaps thousands, of problems one could study with this model. After a few weeks of perfusing rat lungs, Jack put an end to my exuberance.

"I want you to stay in your office, stay at your desk, and work on a hypothesis," he said. "*Your* hypothesis."

Day after day, when the other post-docs were working on their research protocols, generating data with the help of the smart CVP technicians, I sat at my old Army surplus desk with a yellow legal pad and pencil. I read papers—Jack's papers, other papers that the lab had recently produced. I wrote down a paragraph of facts and what we knew about X and Y and how these facts needed to be connected with other facts that we thought were important in controlling the workings of the lung circulation. After ten days, between experiments, Jack, in scrubs, would stick his head through the door and cheerfully ask, "So, what is your hypothesis?"

43

I told him, but he shook his head and said, "No, you don't have a hypothesis." I don't remember what the idea had been that I offered as a hypothesis; the point was, it was no good .And he left. This question-and-answer game went on for four weeks and ended with Jack finally accepting my hypothesis. My hypothesis would be resurrected as a potential treatment of patients with severe pulmonary hypertension thirty years later.

Jack completed an engineering degree from MIT before going to med school. Together with Bob Grover, the founder of the CVP lab, he had built a wooden corral high up on Mt. Evans above Denver to study pulmonary hypertension in steers they had purchased at low altitude in Kansas, shipped to Colorado, and then trucked up to 11,000 feet, close to the summit of Mt. Evans. Jack was born in Hazard, Kentucky, not far from the birthplace of Abraham Lincoln, and as the years went by, I came to appreciate his Lincolnesque sense of humor, his storytelling, and his sharp wit. Jack's story needs to be told by somebody else. I owe the man.

The CVP curriculum included "the research talk." There was a talk to be given by one of the post-docs every morning of the week (Monday to Friday) at eight. There were the experiments. There was writing to do. The philosophy was that the new post-doc had to be broken into pieces, particularly the German ones, which then, over two or three years of hard work, would be put back together—the right way. Jack's method was Socratic and not subtle.

One day, a young man whose application for med school had been rejected twice visited Jack. The awkward young fellow—today the word "geek" would perhaps characterize him—sought Jack's advice on how to be successful and how to get accepted into med school. After listening to the young man's story of failed attempts and unrealized hopes, and studying the young fellow's body language, Jack asked, "Do you play piano?"

"Why? No," muttered the young man. "You think that would get me into med school?"

"No," said Jack, "but you could play piano in a whore house—and that experience might get you into med school." He delivered the opinion with a broad grin and a firm Presbyterian handshake.

The CVP faculty liked to play good cop–bad cop with the fresh post-docs. One of the faculty members would demolish the fellow's research talk at the morning conference, and another faculty member would pick up the pieces the next day. I had several failed talks. When a talk had failed with a B– or C rating, one had two weeks to improve it and do it again. The talk had to be worked out on plain white 8 1/2" x11" sheets of paper, so-called "slides" that were inserted at the end of an archaic projection device—an epidiascope—which I had never seen before and never since. The "epi" was a monstrous metal box with a strong lens, a mirror, a light bulb, and a rubberized conveyor belt that transported the sheet of paper to the center of the gizmo.

The first slide was the title of the talk, the second had to be the hypothesis, and the third gave the rationale for the hypothesis. When the CVP lab faculty had a good day and the big boys were particularly animated, it could happen that the speaker would be interrupted as the hypothesis slide was fed into the epi: "Let me stop you right there," someone would shout. "I don't like your hypothesis!" Or the talk would be stopped at projection slide number three: "This rationale is not anything you can stand on. It's more like quicksand...." Nobody came to the defense of the speaker; he had to get his spirits up and try to tough it out.

Only when I witnessed that invited guest speakers received the same treatment did I warm up to this style of scientific discourse.

Later, the real importance of having a hypothesis was explained to me. If the data failed to support the hypothesis but the hypothesis was specific enough, and the research question was important, then the paper was publishable, and one had only to insert the word "not" into the title of the manuscript. For example:" The number of red blood cells impacts on the pulmonary artery pressure". In fact the number of red cells does affect the lung vascular pressure---so no need here for the "not". Those were the days when one could still publish negative studies if the hypothesis was good.

Through the years, I appreciated Jack's approach, and I understood the meaning of Albert Einstein's statement about the enabling quality of the hypothesis: "Only the hypothesis enables you to see what can be seen."

Without the conceptual framework, data remain just data, and the dots cannot be connected. I also eventually realized that a hypothesis is a challenge to the community of researchers; it can be falsified and proven wrong. If confirmed, it can be amended, expanded, and used to engulf earlier sub-hypotheses. As I think back, I realize how much I owe this man. His one-liners echo in my brain: "Randomize the first patient! To treatment!" "If you don't try, you can't fail." "You could be right about this—but perhaps not." Jack never retired and continued his Socratic teaching until he tragically died—he did not see the oncoming car that ran into him and his bicycle.[27]

---

27 L.G. Moore and R.F. Grover, "Jack Reeves and His Science," Physiol Neurobiology (2006).

Chapter 7

Flat Screens

Usually on Mondays, my office computer would not work. Whatever I tried—shutting it down, rebooting—nothing worked. I could not open my e-mail. I would get an error message that said, "Internet Explorer cannot display the webpage."

When I called the help desk, I would hear this recorded message: "Thank you for calling the Technology Help Desk. All of our service personnel are helping other callers. Your call may be audited. Please stay on the line. Your call is very important to us! Did you know that the hospital is a non-smoking facility? Smoking is bad for your health. If you are pregnant, you should not smoke! Our early-pregnancy health program can be assessed by dialing.... Please stay on the line!"

Some kind of music...

A female voice chirped: "It is the flu season! Don't get sick. Be prepared. Get vaccinated and drink plenty of fluids."

Different music....

"Please stay on the line! Our high blood pressure and stroke prevention program has been designed by some of the best doctors in America. We provide tomorrow's care today."

First kind of music again....

For some years now, I have had vivid fantasies of the future of medicine. I envisioned tomorrow's care to be something like this: The patient arrives in the Emergency Department and is entered into the Total Body Scanner (TBS). The digitalized scans are entered into a database. While this happens, a wine glass full of blood is drawn and sent to the lab. No form needs to be filled out because the lab will test for everything. The lab abnormalities are entered into the database and are analyzed together with the scanned images. As the patient is transported to a hospital room, all the data have been processed, culminating in a list of diagnoses and matching treatments that appear on a flat screen in the patient's room. No caregiver is within sight. As the flat-screen image fades out, a lecture announcement takes shape: "Health care disparities and racial medical issues in American health care," the announcement says. "Today at noon in the Learning Center."

As the team of three doctors enters the patient's room, all armed with handheld computer phones, the team leader, in her mid-thirties, introduces herself to the patient. There are no white doctor coats; they had been banned a long time ago, once the hospital infection control people had found out that bacteria were transported on rounds from one patient to another by the coats.

Then I had a flashback. I remembered how my first steps on the way to become a medical doctor had taken me on the ward of the city hospital in Bayreuth, in Franconia, Germany. I had just finished high school (actually the school was a "gymnasium," the traditional institution that prepares students for the university. The German educational system has no "college." The kids have to know what they want to do and want to be at age eighteen or nineteen). In the hot summer of 1965, I signed up for two months of work in that hospital before medical school classes would start in November.

The cheerful greeting of "Hi, Mr. Washington. We have looked at your data" from the pulmonary fellow brought me back into the twenty-first century.

I was an attending physician on the "consult service"—without a tie (also identified as a bacteria transport vehicle), and Mr. Washington was my patient. "We will have to take a look around your lungs," the fellow began. "This is called a bronchoscopy. We use a flexible light tube, a bit thinner than my pinky, and we may take a little bit of tissue so we can send it to the lab. You have a few nodules in your lung." She took a quarter out of her pocket and added, "One of the nodules is that big. You have been smoking for quite a few years—if this is cancer, the oncologist wants to know your total genome sequencing study, and some microchip studies will tell us about a few genes of interest and several classes of drugs that you will not tolerate."[28]

---

28 Nagrath, et al., "Isolation of Rare Circulating Tumour Cells in Cancer Patients by Microchips Technology," Nature, 450, no. 1235 (2007).

The resident stared at her handheld flat screen and calculated the potential risk of chest surgery, the cost of chemo, and the reimbursement rate of the total hospitalization and procedure costs.

- Lung cancer in the second decade of the twenty-first century continues to be lethal, with a short survival time after diagnosis for most patients. Lung cancer is now the leading cause of cancer death in men and women in America, even though most people have never heard of it.[29] Since 1987, lung cancer has surpassed breast cancer in American women.[30] Annually, 72,000 women die from breast cancer. Between 1930 and 1997, the death rate from lung cancer in women increased by 600 percent. About 25 percent of the women in the United States still smoke, and 50,000 teenage girls smoke.

Mr. Washington was visibly scared and said, "My dad had colon cancer and had surgery, and he is now seventy-six...."

I forgot how many times during my practice I had to sit down with patients and their wives (previously mostly men developed lung cancer; that has now changed) and tell them that the diagnosis was lung cancer. I had not taken an active research interest in lung cancers and had concluded that the reason these cancers were refractory to chemotherapy was the fact that the tumor cells had been selected as survivors of the constant cigarette smoke toxin barrage; the lung cancer had developed because of the decades-long "cigarette chemotherapy." Because of the terrible lung cancer chemotherapy statistics, I saw my role as a doctor at the end of the moment-of-truth conversation with the patient as being that of an end-of-life counselor.

I usually said something like, "it's time to get your house in order— and if you ever wanted to go fishing in Alaska, now is the time to do it," I

29 L.A. Gillman, et al., "NIH Disease Funding Levels and Burden of Disease," PLoS ONE (2011) be16837.
30 K. Pirie, R. Peto, G.K. Reeves, et al., "The 21st Century Hazards of Smoking and Benefitsof Stopping: A Prospective Study of One Million Women in the UK." Lancet (October 26, 2012).

simply was and am a therapeutic nihilist when it comes to advanced lung cancer.

Detection of early lung cancer is quite a different matter. Computed tomography of the chest (CT scanning) now has been shown to detect small tumors that can be surgically resected at a time when there is no metastasis[31.]

One of the very first patients I ever encountered as a pre-med student during that hot summer in the Bavarian city hospital was a man in his early sixties with metastatic lung cancer. The physician I was shadowing had the patient take off his shirt and sit on a gurney. He percussed the thorax of the patient, quickly tapping up and down on the left side of his back as he asked, "You are getting short of breath again?" The patient only nodded as the doctor scrubbed the back with an iodine-dripping sponge. The doctor opened a steel box containing sterilized instruments and filled a syringe with lidocaine. "OK, you know the drill," he said. He pierced the sharp needle at the end of the syringe into the patient's iodined skin between two ribs—"Just a little bee sting"—and the lidocaine was generously injected as the needle probed deeper into the chest wall. As the needle/cannula pierced the chest wall and amber-color fluid gushed out of the chest into the glass container, I passed out. Was it the smell of iodine, the sparkle of the steel cannula? I will never know. Once the container was filled with a liter and a half of this fluid and only a few drops came out of the patient's chest, the man started to cough. The doctor removed the cannula, placed a Band-Aid over the puncture site, and sent the patient home.

So many years later, I can still remember the entire scenario—the patient, the glass cylinder, the orange-brown warm fluid—perhaps because I passed out, perhaps because the doctor was kind enough to say, "Don't worry. This once happened to me too. You will be OK." Metastatic lung cancer is still untreatable today.

We have a breast cancer lobby, "Run for the Cure" events, and an ovarian cell cancer campaign. In some hotels, you find pledge cards on the nightstand that say, "Donate to support breast cancer research." No such lobby exists for lung cancer, which remains in the closet because it is mainly caused by smoking. Lung cancer and smoking: This hypothesis

---

31 Goulart, B.H., et al. J Natl Compr Canc. Netw 10, no. 2 (2012) 267-75.

was first formulated in 1912 [32,] and smoking and lung cancer were experimentally linked for the first time in 1950. The tobacco industry continues to ignore the epidemiological and experimental evidence and ridiculously points out that year-long exposure of mice to tobacco smoke causes some structural upper airway abnormalities—but not lung cancer—which, of course, illustrates that quite frequently the mouse is not a suitable model of human disease. And it is true that there are patients who develop lung cancer without ever having smoked a single cigarette. It is also true that, on the other hand, smoking increases the risk for the development of other cancers—for example, bladder cancer.

It is time for a national lung cancer campaign to raise awareness, to increase research efforts, and to destigmatize the disease. Currently, the research funding is $23,754 per breast cancer death, but only $1,414 per lung cancer death. Two decades ago, psychiatric illnesses were closeted. Now mood disorders have been recognized as potentially treatable illnesses, and several drugs are on the market. Every effort should be made to identify patients at risk for developing lung cancer. We are not good at making an early diagnosis of lung cancers. Frequently, a routine chest x-ray finds a lung lesion that is worked up, revealing the cancer diagnosis after a biopsy. A blood test is needed, and people at risk need to be frequently screened; their lungs need to be imaged serially. After all, we use mammograms for breast cancer screening. One can easily start with multiyear smokers who have a family history of any cancer. If the father of the patient and two uncles had a cancer, the risk of a smoker to develop a tobacco-related malignancy is clearly higher. A family like that harbors a cancer gene or several cancer genes. Emphysema also increases the risk of lung cancer. And then there is the principle of chemoprevention. Could aspirin reduce the risk of lung cancer as it reduces the risk of colon cancer?

We need bright daylight on lung cancer to make it a preventable and treatable disease.

The thoracocentesis (draining of the pleural fluid) that I had witnessed until I fainted in the hospital in Bayreuth so many years ago is still performed today when the metastases in the epithelial cells lining the lung release growth factors that make the lung tissue leaky. It is part of palliative lung cancer care.

---

32 L. Adler, Primary Malignant Growth of the Lungs and Bronchi (London: Longmans,– Green and Company, 1912).

Chapter 8

Clinician–Scientists and Translational Research

The formerly legendary chiefs of medicine departments at many univer-sities in the United States accomplished the goal to build their depart-ments around "clinician–scientists" or "clinician–investigators." They were quite successful in filling the endocrinology–rheumatology–infectious dis-eases divisions with such physicians. They often were or became members of the American Society of Clinical Investigation, the "young Turks" who published their papers in the Society's prestigious journal, the *Journal of Clinical Investigation*. These individuals had research grants that allowed them to reduce their clinical service time and permitted them to run a lab. That's the way it was. During the many years of taking care of patients, I never had any doubts that understanding the pathophysiology, the sys-tematic investigation of what goes wrong in disease, the mechanisms of disease ,was the only way to make progress in medicine.

About to graduate from the German high school, my father had asked me what I would want to do for a living after graduation, and I offered him a catalog of subjects to study at the university, starting with biochemistry and German literature and ending with architecture. I offered everything except medicine. He finally asked, "Why would you not consider medical school?" There I was at the dinner table, and an answer was required. After all, my father would be the one paying for my education.

"Yes," I said reluctantly, "if this does not automatically mean for you that I take over your practice…." I knew my dad would be upset hearing this, but I just could not say, "Yes, I will consider medicine," giving him the impression that I would at some time continue his work in his general internal medicine practice in the small county seat in northeastern Bavaria. I had grown up with "the practice." My parents' house was an extension of the doctor's office. The doctor's office was connected with the main hallway of our house, and the basement had been covered with lead-containing plaster to safely house the x-ray machine. Growing up, I had my chest x-ray taken and played with the heavy, lead-enforced leather glove that my father put on his right hand before touching a patient when the rays were on.

I remember the Abbot of a small monastery, Father Basileus, in his brown monk's habit, complete with a white rope belt, rotund and smiling through his gold-rimmed glasses, sitting in our entrance hall waiting for the results of his blood sugar test. Private patients did not enter through the office door but through the house door, and they did not have to wait in the common patients' waiting room. Because Father Basileus had traveled from his monastery on an empty stomach, he received breakfast, prepared by my mother, after his blood test. I watched how he moved a breakfast roll and cooked ham around on his plate—the authentic image of the medieval brewer monk on Bavarian beer bottles. For sure, that was personalized medicine.

I remember answering our doorbell at seven in the morning to find a patient who asserted, "I am on my way to work. I thought I could pick up my prescriptions."

Back at the dinner table, my dad was deeply upset. "So what kind of medicine do you have in mind?"

Of course I had no idea. I just knew that I could not be a country doctor taking care of patients with back pain and diabetes who would knock at the door at seven in the morning asking for their prescriptions. I do remember that it was the daily routine that I feared. I had already noted my dad's frustration with patients' wear-and-tear problems and his unsuccessful strategies aimed to convince his patients of necessary lifestyle changes.

When I mumbled that I wanted to test drugs in animals, he concluded, "So, you want to become a rat doctor!"

He was right. My first experimental animals were inbred white rats with red eyes, and even after years, my father never really made peace with my choice of a career to become a clinician–scientist.

A recent editorial states that about 2 percent of the physicians in the United States are "physician–scientists." So what is a physician–scientist? My own definition of this profession is a physician who does the work that is done neither by the basic researcher (basic biomedical scientists explore the crystal structure of molecules and figure out what they do, and among many other things, they identify new targets for drugs) nor by the mainstream clinician. He is a physician who is not satisfied with knowing "what to do"; he needs to know how things work and why they work.

This point was brought to my clear attention many years ago, one Sunday morning on rounds in the intensive care unit. As the on-call resident presented a case of diabetic ketoacidosis (a dangerous form of diabetic coma in which the blood and cells become acidic), I had fallen into my usual teaching mode, asking the team why the kidney function was compromised in diabetic ketoacidosis. The resident interrupted me coldly and said, "Please don't tell me how it works—just tell me what to do!"

Don't tell us how things go wrong. I was speechless for a moment. I had forgotten that treatment algorithms and practice guidelines had become important topics on teaching rounds. It had never occurred to me that one could teach "what to do" without teaching "how it works." I thought that was not an option for academic teachers.

I had already found out that the physician–scientist sits uncomfortably between the chairs, not fully accepted by the molecular biochemist and watched suspiciously by the full-blooded clinician. The basic scientist would say, when times get tough and funding for research dries up, "You can always make a living seeing patients—I cannot." And the clinician will say, with some justification, "Just because it works in your rats means nothing for my patients." This always made it very clear: *my* rats, *her* patients—as if I did not have my own patients who were dying from a rare lung disorder.

This decade-old debate about clinical research pitted against basic research goes on in academic institutions, and once a year, in certain journals, an established and well-funded investigator deplores the situation of the physician–scientist, characterizing such a person as a member of an endangered species.[33] "Please, protect the clinician–scientist," the authors write. "Let us invest in 'translational research,'" they say. New drug treatment is needed—not only to fuel the pharmaceutical industry."

Several years ago, the National Institutes of Health (NIH) developed a road map for what is now called "translational medicine." The slogan

---

33 R.G. Khadaroo, and O.D. Rotstein, "Are Clinician–Scientists an Endangered Species? Barriers to Clinician–Scientist Training," Clin Invest Med 25, no. 6 (2002): 260–1.

"From the bench to the bedside" became popular. Having one foot in the clinic and the other in a lab requires the constant shuttling from one to the other. This requires one to have and maintain a research lab and to finance it. This means having access to patients, and they are frequently sequestered by *"my patient"* clinicians, who will cheerfully pronounce, "She who controls the patients controls the agenda and the budget."

Prior to the bust of the economic bubble in 2008, the NIH road map called for the development of Centers for Translational Research (CFTRs) and provided money as an incentive. Research buildings were built, and directors of some fifty CFTRs were named. They hired administrators and statisticians, and they now provide core services. What remains unclear today is whether this infrastructure investment has really improved the work of physician–scientists, has produced an increased number of new junior physician–scientists, or has turned out to be another example of failed trickle-down economics. It is more likely that the fight for survival of a physician–investigator and his or her lab in "this economy"[34] is more desperate than ever before. The translational medicine bridge is spanning a deep and wide chasm where clinical trialists on one side control their patients to protect them from participating in innovative studies and where basic scientists in grant-review committees are shooting applications down while cheerfully shouting, "No mouse, no money!" (Meaning: "Your work is pedestrian without a genetically engineered mouse model.") With the CFTRs, we have many new school buses and bus drivers. But what if the seats in the buses remain empty?

As the competition for the shrinking research budget gets fiercer, the "spirit of translation" has become merely an afterthought, not the driving force for new developments. On the one side, we have expensive big pharma trials, and on the other side, we have gene knockouts in mice that produce phenotypes in search of human diseases. Highly necessary pre-clinical studies—which should move experimental drugs to rapid clinical application—are being conducted using animal models that frequently do

---

34 S.F. Roberts, et al., "Perspective: Transforming Science into Medicine: How Clinician–Scientists Can Build Bridges across Research's 'Valley of Death,'" *Academic Medicine*, 87, no. 3 (2012): 266–70.

not represent the salient features of the target human disease. Why this disconnect?

It is easier to test new drugs using old and inadequate animal models than it is to build disease-relevant new models. Building new models is part of the job of the physician–investigator.

Step one: She observes patients and studies a disease and then develops a hypothesis that can explain the main hallmarks of the disease.

Step two: She tests the hypothesis, which requires the building of new animal models. These models should reproduce predictably the major components of the disease and allow the study of disease progression and the dissection of disease mechanisms on the level of tissues and the involved cells.

> Step three: She tests in these disease-relevant models how disease development (called pathogenesis) can be prevented and how the established disease can be treated effectively. And, of course, the cure can't be worse than the disease.

Thousands of very sophisticated research papers in addition to numerous practice guidelines are published every year, but the clinical success is meager. Not enough of the basic science data change our clinical practice. Progress is slow.

There is another problem: It has become nearly impossible to publish negative data. This is bad because we should not forget that the patient is the center of all of this research.

And another issue: Many of the engineered models make one point and one point only. The value of this point is unclear when the experts only reluctantly acknowledge the model's limitations. Many pre-clinical animal endpoints do not use clinically meaningful predicative biomarkers. We are now obsessed with mechanistic endpoints, to the point where it almost does not matter whether a drug or treatment works. If a treatment works, but we do not completely understand the mechanism of action, the experiments or studies are often dismissed as "pure phenomenology." "Descriptive research" is the curse word of the day, the death sentence for many grant applications. Of course, we prefer to know how a particular treatment works, but occasionally we will have to move forward without having an exact mechanism of drug action. We have prescribed aspirin for eighty years and treated many pains without understanding its precise molecular mechanism of action.

Perhaps the clinician–scientist, that always-endangered species, will eventually become extinct. Some people do research so that they can write a grant, and other people write a grant so they can do research. Then who is to blame? The economy? The market? Perhaps it will become necessary for medical schools, in their curricula, to make an effort and begin to put a new focus on "Tell me how it works," "It works—but we don't understand why!" and "Why don't we have any drugs to treat this disease?"

I sometimes think it is curious that if we have a patient who speaks only Chinese, we ask for a translator. But when it comes to complex human diseases, we think we can do without a translator. The paradigm shift of translational medicine will require a new infrastructure and a change of culture. Academic institutions can incentivize clinicians to ask for the translator. A conference room, somewhere between the lab and the ward, would be neutral ground, where the two worlds of basic and clinical research could meet. The deans of medical schools could provide "glue grants" to finance the critically important pilot projects. Such measures could amount to a climate change in medicine.

Chapter 9

High Colonics, Magnetic Water, and the "Art of Medicine"

The lab meeting was over when my cell phone rang the aria of the "Queen of Night" from Mozart's *Magic Flute*. It was John telling me, with pauses between short sentences, that Susan had died that morning. He had checked on her at 3:30, and she was OK; when he checked again around 4:30, she was not breathing. When my wife and I had told him two weeks before that Susan was in the "home stretch," he had said, "Perhaps a few more months." But he had listened to us, and the day after our last visit with Susan, he had arranged for home hospice.

That night, two weeks earlier, we had all been together. My wife, the orthopedic surgeon, had turned into little Red Riding Hood and brought a basket with food and a bottle of champagne. Susan was giddy and high as a kite on steroids. This usually so-quiet woman would not stop talking. The bone mets (metastases) were not a problem now—it was her liver that was filled with them. She hardly sipped from the Kir Royale that John had made and talked about that large clock that she wanted to have in her room "The hands should be two feet long so I can see the time." And she liked the cannabis because it made everything more real: "You know, there are few things more real than stage four cancer." She laughed and said she felt so sensuous. The logs in the kiva fireplace sent some sparks into the cold winter night. John refrained from joking, yet there still was his upside-down-hanging Christmas tree—"My Baselitz tree," he said. He had some of Susan's large water-color landscapes up in the gallery, and Susan said that her last painting was the red brushstroke on this year's Christmas card—a single large, vibrating stroke that fizzled out toward the bottom of the card. She said that now she understood things better and explained the large painting of Francis Bacon in the book she leafed through as "Van Gogh showing up for work."[35]It was one of several of Bacon's Van Gogh's paintings in rather ghoulish colors: Vincent under a tree, satchel on his back. "Francis Bacon had meant to show Vincent going out for the last time on the day he shot himself;you see, I know this now", Susan said.

Susan had detected the cancer herself. At that time, thirteen of fifteen nodes were positive. The oncologist said, "We can try some radiation." At that time, I worked at the University of Colorado as a pulmonologist (lung doctor). John, my friend, was despondent as he told me over the phone, "Breast cancer, positive nodes, they want to radiate."

It took me a few seconds before I yelled "Malpractice!" into the phone. Then I said, "You guys have to come to Denver and see the breast cancer team at the university."

A week later, John and Susan drove up from New Mexico. Susan got her second opinion and was directed to heavy-duty chemotherapy, followed by bone marrow transplantation using her own marrow. She got the chemo, lost her hair, got the bone marrow, and everything went swimmingly. After four weeks, they drove back down to God's country unconvinced that she had had a successful treatment. The tumor had been positive for estrogen receptors, and she took tamoxifen[36] or several years. She had one bout of lung injury following her transplant, and it was successfully treated with steroids. That was it. That was twelve years ago. She was OK. Back to normal life, traveling, painting in Venice, more hair than ever before.

Susan was OK. A few years ago, she complained about shoulder pain, a rotator cuff injury. Of course she found someone to operate, but she was not better afterward. Other than that, she was doing everything she liked to do until in the late fall two years ago, she felt weak all of a sudden and had muscle pain all over—some kind of flu, John diagnosed.

"Any fever, a cough, the sniffles?" I asked.

"No" was the answer.

Blood tests were done; one showed that an enzyme, alkaline phosphatase, was about tenfold higher than normal. A month went by. Every medical student could connect the dots: history of breast cancer + pain +

---

35 Based on Van Gogh's 1888 oil The Painter on the Road to Tarascon.
36 Tamoxifen and chemotherapy interact in patients with node-negative, estrogen recep-tor-positive breast cancer.

elevated alkaline phosphatase = bone metastases, until proven otherwise. A computed tomography (CT scan) study showed many bone lesions, and the local medical environment recommended "hospice and oxycontin."

The doctors at the Breast Cancer Center at Denver thought otherwise and moved ahead with nuclear medicine. They were treating Susan with a bone-seeking radioactive emitter (both photon and positron emitters are used) and gave her a survival time of around two years.

After the treatment in Denver had been completed and after her return to the mountains of northern New Mexico, she and John fell under the spell of a local self-appointed "healer," and this is what the final phase of this story is about.

When my orthopedic surgeon wife inquired whether Susan received follow-up care by the doctors at the Breast Cancer Center at Anschutz in Denver, her husband John said, "No, but Joseph is taking care of her."

Who on God's earth was Joseph, and what did he do? Reluctantly, John doled out information one piece at a time. A comfortable chair had been moved downstairs. That is where Joseph would do the infusions. Infusions of what? By a man who was not even a licensed nurse. And apparently day after day. When we heard this, my wife and I were upset and furious, and we said so. There was the specter of infection, sepsis, and endocarditis (infection of heart valves). But there was more.

There was "magnetic' water,"[37,38], and there were "high colonics" and steroids—a complete treatment plan that also included intravenous vitamin C and the blood thinner heparin.[39]

---

37 "Imagination without magnetism produces convulsions; magnetism without imagination produces nothing." Jean Silviain Bailly
38 Magnetism was practiced by the French physician Anton Mesmer. Later on, the German-born physicist Klaus Kronenberg, who died at the age of 86 in California and had worked for the Magnetics Company in Valpariso, Indiana, became a proponent of magne-tizing water. Kronenberg taught that water in a magnetic fieldwill change its properties. For example calcium carbonate will precipitate in the form of aragonite (named after the Molinda de Aragon in Spain). Imbibing of magnetic water is supposed to reduce the "acidity of the body," "regulate blood and red blood cell chemistry," and "increase intracellular hydration." Health benefits from drinking magnetic water presumably are reduction of back pain; magnetic water also has been recommended as a treatment of migraines.
39 Fanikos, et al., Amer J Med 124, no. 12, (2011):1143-50.

John paid for the expensive magnetic water (one supplier of magnetic products is Alibaba, a company that also offers magnetic levitation devices) and all the rest of the "do-it-yourself medicine." After getting over my initial anger and disgust, I settled down and reflected on the "treatment" plan. This "do-it-yourselfer" was not entirely ruthless, nor was he stupid. He must have done some reading. He probably had read that there were high-dose vitamin C-infusion trials ongoing and sponsored by the National Cancer Institute. He must have known that massive intravenous vitamin C causes the blood sodium level to rise—that's why he drew blood once a week and sent it to the lab. He also needed to monitor blood coagulation variables and platelet numbers (heparin can decrease the platelet count). But why heparin? To prevent cancer-related thrombosis? Or did he know the Harvard physician's work? Or maybe he knew about Karnofski's publications on heparin-binding growth factors? Or did he follow the heparin-for-cancer debate?[39]

Colonic irrigation. What about that? In the Western world and medicine, "bad humors" have played a big role ever since Hippocrates and Galen. Autointoxiation had been considered a major etiological factor (causing diseases). Autointoxication should not be confused with "autoimmunity," although Paul Ehrlich introduced the idea of antibodies under the rubric of "horror autotoxicus" (fear of self-intoxication). It is true that our immune system can generate antibodies that can be directed against the body's cells, but the proponents of the idea of autointoxication advocate colonic irrigations and coffee enemas. The symptoms of autointoxication include fatigue, depression, poor appetite, and headache. What is most fascinating is that the recent investigations of mucosal immunity and of the gut immune system and the gut biome are providing solid biological information that somewhere intersects and overlaps with the last century theories of Ludwig Brieger and Herman Senator, who apparently identified the chemical processes underlying the intestinal toxin generation.[40]

Czech playwright Vaclav Havel said, as quoted in the obituary by Paul Wilson in the February 9 2012 issue of the *New York Review of Books*, "Hope

---

39 E.A. Akl, and H.J. Schunemann, "Routine Heparin for Patients with Cancer?One Answer, More Questions," New England Journal of Medicine 366, no. 7 (2012): 661–2.
40 E. Ernst, "Colonic Irrigation and the Theory of Autointoxication: A Triumph of Ignorance over Science," Journal of Clinical Gastroenterology 4 (1997) 196-8.

is not the conviction that something will turn out well, but the certainty that something makes sense, regardless of how it turns out." My oncologist friends had explained to me that patients on a treatment protocol—experimental or not—may do better because they feel more cared for and because the more frequent monitoring of lab values and imaging required by a study protocol can often detect evidence of disease progression. In that scenario, infectious complications can be discovered earlier, and patients may get better pain management. Then there is the placebo effect and, most importantly, patients conclude that they have not given up. There is hope somewhere. Whether or not Joseph's treatment plan prolonged Susan's life or quality of life, we will never know. She lived about as long as the oncologists in Colorado had estimated, based on her disease and the metastatic burden.

Home hospice was not required for Susan for long—just a few days after the infusions had been stopped.

Such is the story of alternative medicine. Growing up in Germany with its spas (a lucrative parallel universe of health care that employs about ten million health care workers and service providers), "healer/practitioners," and concepts of psychosomatic medicine, I have over the years tried to keep an open mind about alternative medicine. My father, who was a general internist and radiologist, often complained about the "healer" in a neighboring town who used a shiny apparatus. Green and red lights would rapidly go on and off after the patient stuck her hand into the dark tunnel at the front end of the gizmo. The "healer" would then read signals emitted from the machine and say, "You have one hundred and forty-four toxins circulating in your blood." Thereafter, an assistant would deliver three elegantly shaped glass vials that contained very bitter-tasting, colored liquids. The healer would then look at the patient and say with the greatest conviction, "This medicine is very new, it is produced in small batches in Switzerland, and it is very expensive." Each of the elements of the formula—new, Switzerland, and expensive—were essential for the treatment success.

A three-month supply of the medicine was mailed to the (usually well-to-do) patient. Upon the patient's return for the follow-up visit, again the diagnosis gizmo flickered, but for a shorter period. The "healer" now could say, "We made significant progress. We are now down to ninety-nine toxins."

In 1998, NIH opened a National Center for Complementary and Alternative Medicine. Its mission is to investigate practices like acupuncture, weird diets, and Chinese herbs and minerals. The institute has a modest budget and keeps a low profile. On the other hand, the industry, which sells vitamin pills, zinc and selenium, and flax seed extracts, has a large advertising budget and is a multibillion-dollar business.

You may wonder where I stand on this. I am with William Osler, Sir William, the patron saint of modern American medicine. He clearly taught both the science and the art of medicine. Before our profession became a job in "an industry like any other industry," doctors had profoundly simple goals: to cure, and if this goal was unattainable, to make the patient feel better.

As Chief Resident, I had the good fortune to work for one year on the private patient ward (then the major source of income of the head of a medicine department at a university hospital in Germany—the patients all had private health insurance in a two-class system of otherwise socialized medicine). To watch the master clinician practice his art was one of the great experiences during my formative years. There would be other role models I remember. I will introduce them later. About halfway through my Chief Resident rotation, which included the requirement to be "on call" all the time, but also to have breakfast with the nurses after we had finished rounding with the Chief. I realized that the professor at the time, before the second world war, as he was my age, had to make do without antibiotics, insulin, and steroids. In his formative years, medicine was largely about making the correct diagnosis, and there were few drugs available to treat diseases. He was a master of the "at first glance" diagnosis, and he was very experienced in the selective use of placebos. A close second to "first, do no harm" (Hippocrates) was "make the patient (feel) better." Like the surgeon's maxim, "A chance to cut is a chance to cure," his maxim was "Almost everything needs to be tried to make the patient better."

That sums it up. The art of medicine is hardly taught anymore today. The art of medicine has been surrendered to practice guidelines and algorithms that are like pinball machines, nervously lighting up and rumbling as the patient is being processed.

Chapter 10

The Respirator: A Device for Prolonging Life—Not Death

It was nighttime in the medical intensive care unit (MICU) of the University Hospital in Hamburg–Eppendorf. I had arrived for my night shift at eight o'clock. For six months, I had worked in this twenty-bed unit and learned how to use the tools of the trade from my older colleagues: how to intubate, how to "put in" a central line, how to deal with a massive gastrointestinal hemorrhage, how to treat a patient who was in a diabetic coma.

During the day, two physicians worked in the MICU, and at night, only one. You were it, and in this case, I was it! The night was warm, some of the windows facing the park were half open, and I could hear the noise of the city. All the patients were tucked in, and it promised to be an uneventful night. But after midnight, we had two back-to-back admissions. One of the patients had been delivered by ambulance with acute chest pain and the diagnosis of acute myocardial infarct; the other patient, in his eighties, was diagnosed with pulmonary edema. While the nurses put the EKG monitor leads on the infarct patient, I gave my full attention to the man in respiratory distress. He was alert and fighting for his next breath. Both of his legs were swollen with edema, and his lips were blue. As the nurses prepared the intubation tray, I stepped out of the unit and found two elderly women who had accompanied the patient on his ambulance ride. They were not relatives; the patient had none. I informed the ladies that I would put a breathing tube into the neck and start mechanical respiration. They nodded approvingly and said, "Mr. Weber is the last butler, the last surviving butler of von Bismarck." They were referring to Otto von Bismarck, 1815–1898[41], the iron chancellor of Wilhelm II, King of Prussia. Indeed,

---

41 Henry Kissinger said, "The man of "blood and iron" wrote prose of extraordinary directness and lucidity comparable in distinctiveness to Churchill's use of the English language."

Mr. Weber had had a pension and continued to live on "the grounds of Friedrichsruh Manor," where the ambulance drivers had picked him up for the straight transport to the University Hospital. A minute later, the patient, still on the gurney, now with rattling breath sounds, faced me as I approached him with the tracheal tube in my hands, and with great effort he said, "I don't think we want to do this." And then he smiled and touched my arm. I put the breathing tube down and suddenly felt loneliness, along with great respect and sadness—all at the same time. "Sir, you are sure?"

"Yes I am sure," he said.

By then, he had intravenous access, and I injected a small dose of morphine. An hour later, the last of Bismarck's butlers had passed away peacefully; he was eighty-five.

The first respirators that were used extensively were the "iron lungs." There was not much of a lung to them but a lot of steel. They were steel tubes into which the patient was inserted with his or her head sticking out. Air was sucked out of the sealed-off steel cylinder with a vacuum pump to expand the patient's lung while the lung collapsed once the tube pressure went to zero, and another vacuum pump pushed air into the tube so that the air was emptied from the lung. The forerunners of the iron lung had been leather and wood bellows.

I remember that my father, as a young doctor practicing medicine at the city hospital of Bayreuth, had picked up patients with polio and paralysis of their respiratory center. He told me that sometimes he had lost the race to the hospital, which had twenty or more of these shiny tubes lined up, row after row, in gym-sized halls.

Bismarck introduced the Health Insurance Bill of 1883. The program was established to provide health care for a large segment of German workers. The employers contributed one-third, and the workers contributed two-thirds of the payment. The minimum payments for medical treatment and sick pay for up to thirteen weeks were legally fixed.

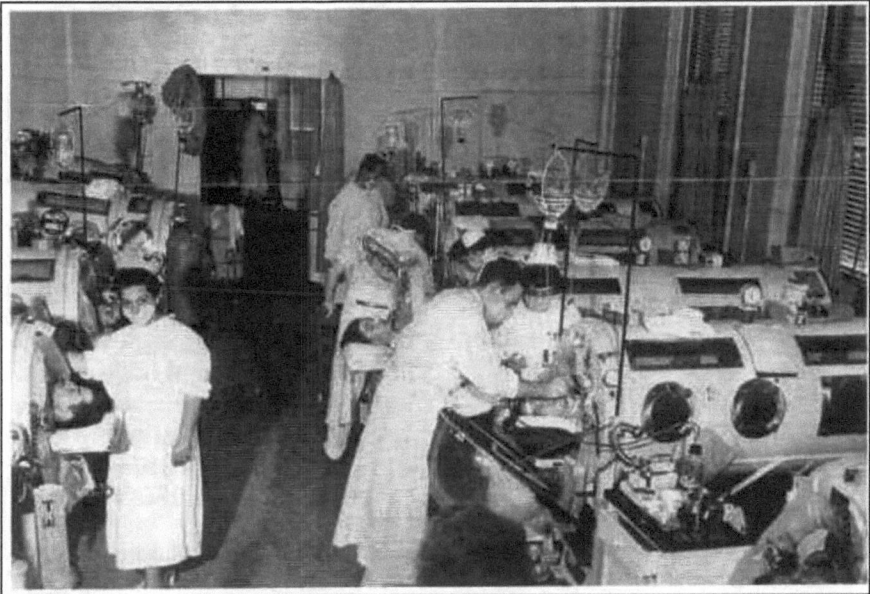

The principle that these mechanical respirators were built on was simple. The rigid steel tube was fixed, and by changing the volume of air in the steel tube, the pressure on the chest wall and on the lungs could be changed rhythmically. The first clinical use of the iron lung, or Drinker Respirator, was in 1928 at the Children's Hospital in Boston. The first patient was an eight-year-old girl with infantile paralysis, or polio. In 1931, John H. Emerson introduced an improved version of this negative-pressure ventilator. One of these machines was used by the patient Barton Herbert from Covington, Louisiana, until his death in 2003 and then was donated to the Centers for Disease Control and Prevention Museum. Interestingly enough, as late as 2008, these iron lungs were still used by a small number of patients. A patient died in 2009 in Australia after having used the iron lung for more than sixty years. See the photo[42]

During my pulmonary fellowship training in Colorado, I got to know a woman who used a negative-pressure cuirass ventilator—an upper-body

---

42 The figurewas reproduced from J.A. Hobin and R.A. Galbraith, "Engaging Basic Scientists in Translational Research," FASEB 26 (2012): 2227.

shell that we called "turtle shell"—for treatment of her post-polio respiratory syndrome.

The British engineer Roger Manley developed a ventilator, the Manley Mark II, and Forrest Bird developed a small green box called the "Bird. Thereafter, positive-pressure ventilation spread quickly. In 1971, Elema–Schölander developed the first Servo ventilator.

Nowadays, ventilators are programmable, computerized machines that allow various modes of ventilation and provide real-time graphical display of volume and pressure curves and allow the calculation of a number of variables like minute ventilation and peak airway pressure.

Taking care of patients with lung diseases includes ventilator support in the intensive care units. Mechanical ventilation was and is guided by measurement of the partial pressure of blood oxygen and carbon dioxide. This requires an arterial blood sample obtained by puncture of an artery or squeezed out of an earlobe in the form of arterialized blood. A low level of arterial oxygen pressure means that a patient is not well oxygenated, and a high level of carbon dioxide means that a patient is not well ventilated. In any case, the ventilator has to be adjusted. In the MICU in Hamburg–Eppendorf, the doctor on call would measure the "blood gases," operating a tricky Radiometer machine based on the principle of Schollander. Fine, long capillary glass tubes were filled with the patient's blood, which was aspirated into a measuring chamber; before that, the device had to be equilibrated against a standard gas provided from a metal gas bottle. In the Denver hospitals, blood-gas technicians measured the blood gases throughout the night. The technicians were ordered to call the pulmonary fellow after each sample had been measured. A fellow found out whether he or she was disliked when called every hour or liked when the technician would bundle the results from several patients to call once or twice during the night. This way, the pulmonary fellow followed each of the ventilated patients in the hospital and knew when to get up from the cot in the call room and adjust the ventilator. The experience with ventilated patients thus accumulated by a pulmonary fellow was substantial.

I also quickly learned that it was easy to start mechanical ventilation but occasionally highly challenging to wean patients off mechanical ventilation. During the first day of my rotation as a pulmonary fellow through the University Hospital, I was asked to see a twenty-year-old patient who had developed ARDS (Adult Respiratory Distress Syndrome, originally described by Tom Petty, my division head) following a liver transplant. Those were the early days of liver transplant and respiratory care. The young woman had been ventilated and successfully weaned off from ventilation, but later on she developed pneumonia and ARDS for a second time. When I saw her, it was six months after her surgery. She was in a small, single-bed room on the transplant ward and ventilated through a tracheostomy tube. She was malnourished, weak, and miserable. The job at hand was to wean her off the ventilator. After one week of efforts that frustrated the patient and me, I probed the lower ranks of the surgery residents to find out whether the Chief of Surgery would consider a transfer to medicine, to the MICU. "We are just better staffed and can spend more time," I said. The mighty Chief consented, and Cherryl became a medicine patient. She was placed in a large corner room of the MICU that had large windows—a contrast to her previous dungeon.

Soon the weaning team, "the weaners," went to work. A half-inch corrugated plastic piece of tubing was connected to the tracheostomy tube, and a large earpiece, which was connected to a Hewlett-Packard oxymeter the size of a carry-on suitcase, was strapped around her ear. The T-piece tubing delivered humidified air. Cherryl was comfortably sitting in a recliner, and the ventilator was shut off. She would breathe on her own for a couple of minutes, turn blue, and everybody would freak out. Back on the blower.

The weaning trials were conducted four times per day. Cherryl, always in her chair, now predictably turned blue after a few minutes and was quickly put back on the ventilator. The question became: can't or won't? She was a bit stronger now, not infected, had no fever, was eating, there was no obvious reason. She was not anemic.

I watched the respiratory nurses from outside the room putting the T-piece on the tracheostomy tube and the oxygen monitor on her ear. Cherryl could watch the number on the instrument. Finally, I figured it out: She had learned that the oxygen saturation number dropped rapidly if she took a series of shallow breaths. As the oxygen saturation fell below 70 percent, the alarm went off, and she was again connected to the machine. Cherryl was in control of this weaning protocol.

I concluded that she did not want to come off of the ventilator. As I shared my conclusion with the seasoned "weaners," we all started to talk about what to do next. One of the technicians, with a big smile, suggested: "We can take her across the street to the CI" (College Inn), a bar that I knew from Friday happy hours.

The next day at noon, we packed Cherryl into a wheelchair and connected her to a battery-powered small ventilator—"the Bird." We told her that we would all join her in an "outing." One respiratory technician, two nurses, I, the pulmonary first-year fellow; we all headed for the elevator down to the main entrance, across Ninth Avenue and into the smoke-filled CI. We put Cherryl at the head of the table; the nurses pulled their Marlboros out and lit up. Then they asked, "Cherryl, what would you like to drink?"

She mouthed, "Gin fizz!"

We all laughed, and she got her drink.

As I escorted the patient back to the hospital across Ninth Avenue, it finally occurred to me that this outing had not been sanctioned by anyone and that a bad outcome would have gotten us all in deep trouble. That afternoon, we resumed the weaning, and this time Cherryl worked with us. The spell was broken—no more shallow breaths. Two weeks later, she was discharged home, after seven months in the hospital.

I always thought Colorado's capital was more than a cow town, but the cow town side of Denver in those days was highlighted every January at the time of the Stockshow. The Stockshow swept groomed heifers and their rancher owners from Montana, Wyoming, Nebraska, and Kansas into the coliseum for the rodeo and the barrel-riding contests. High school girls proudly polished their pet goats to high sheen, and the parents were proud of their kids. On Friday afternoon of the first Stockshow weekend, a fifty-eight-year-old rancher from Cheyenne, Wyoming, was admitted to the MICU with "respiratory distress." He was one of those tough, skinny, frontiersmen. The nurses observed that his behind was too small for his jeans as they peeled him out of them. His breathing was visibly labored; he was sitting up, resting on his arms to catch his breath. He was barrel-chested and had big-time emphysema. He was put on high-flow oxygen delivered via a face mask. As his respiratory rate bumped up to thirty-six, he was intubated.

A few hours went by, and, like the "Queen of the Night" of *Mozart's Magic Flute*, the rancher's wife arrived to set the MICU team straight and to threaten everyone involved in Jeremy's care. Everything was piercing about this woman: her glance, her voice, her elbows. She was dressed for the Stockshow, wearing cowboy boots and a flannel shirt with mother of pearl buttons. A bandanna was wrapped around her neck.

"What the hell is going on here? My husband never wanted to be on a ventilator—and he is not going to be. I want him off this damn machine!"

"Does your husband have an advance directive or living will?" I asked.

"No, he doesn't, and we don't think about this kind of nonsense."

Battle-hardened after years in the ICU, I searched for a strategy to win the "Queen of the Night" over. I knew I needed to be patient. I started to explain that her husband had pneumonia, which we believed would respond to antibiotic treatment, and that the pneumonia compromised a lung that was already quite damaged by more than forty years of smoking cigarettes. I explained that mechanical ventilation was life saving and, we hoped, temporary.

"Jeremy never wanted to be hooked up to a machine!" she screamed.

"If we take him off the ventilator, your husband is going to die," I said.

"How do you know this? And how long do you plan to play this ventilator game?" Clearly, the rancher's wife was not passive-aggressive; she was furious and impossible to deal with.

"That is what I want to talk with you about next. My plan is to do a tracheostomy—tomorrow. This will allow us to start weaning him off the machine much earlier. In fact," I said, "this is the only way we will get him off the machine." I thought about something Dr. T.L. Petty, my division head and the world-famous chair of the Pulmonary and Critical Care Medicine division at the University of Colorado Medical Sciences Center, had said: "The respirator is a device for prolonging life—not death."

I asked whether there were other family members in town, and reluctantly she admitted that her son and daughter were also in Denver. I proposed a family meeting for the next day. Family dynamics in the ICU environment at the time of death and dying are often the deciding issue, and there are big cultural and ethnic differences; fundamentally there is the issue of trust.

The next morning, the patient's wife and adult son and daughter appeared—one hour after the appointed time. I collected the nurses taking care of Jeremy, the ICU charge nurse, and a seasoned respiratory nurse, and we sat down in the MICU conference room.

To be on the safe side, I started out with this question: "Who is your spokesperson?" and to my big surprise, as the "queen" was taking a big breath to launch her speech, the son said calmly, "Mother, let me handle this!" Mother became red-faced, got up, and stormed out of the conference room. The son listened to my explanation of why a tracheostomy would facilitate weaning—the patient can eat, he is easier to mobilize (he can sit in a comfortable chair), bronchodilator drugs can be administered directly into the airways—and he agreed to the procedure. But the patient's wife was the decision maker. It was Saturday, so members of the hospital's ethics committee were not available, and a court-appointed guardianship was a remote theoretical possibility. I had called the ENT (ear, nose, and throat) doctor to be available and to get the consent form for the tracheostomy signed by the "queen." We started paging her over the hospital's intercom system. Mrs..., please return to the Medical Intensive Care Unit." It took her an hour, but finally she came back.

"Please sit down with the ENT doctor; he will explain the procedure, the risks, and benefits." Another half hour went by; she signed the consent form, and we rolled Jeremy into the operating room.

The story ended well. Jeremy's pneumonia responded to the antibiotics. Short weaning periods were tolerated, he sat in the chair and read the newspaper that his children had brought, and soon he required ventilator support only through the night. Then the respirator was unhooked, and oxygen was delivered directly through the tracheal tube that by now was a "talking" tube; Jeremy was eating well, ambulating, and getting his strength back. Finally, the trach tube was pulled, and he walked out of the MICU escorted by son and daughter and cheered on by the nurses.

The wife was nowhere to be seen. Perhaps she had returned to Cheyenne to take care of the animals.

Chapter 11

More Important than Pain: The Desire to Be in Control

Tom Petty—not the rock star, but the chair of the Pulmonary and Critical Care Medicine division at the University of Colorado Medical Sciences Center—was world-famous. He had put the syndrome of acute respiratory failure in adults on the map. He and his colleagues produced a milestone medical paper that was rejected by fourteen medical journals before its final acceptance and publication in the British *Lancet*. Tom succeeded Roger Mitchell, who was a TB (tuberculosis) doctor with an early keen interest in emphysema and COPD (chronic pulmonary obstructive disease). Both Roger and Tom were outstanding clinicians, but it was Tom Petty who had the vision of what modern pulmonary medicine would look like in the post-tuberculosis area. He also accepted the responsibility to implement his vision by building the Denver Pulmonary Medicine training program. Tom was impressive as a teacher, and he led by example.

That prompts me to elaborate a bit about these very important principles of the patient–physician contract. It's about truth—telling the truth, delivering the bad news, and putting it in perspective. I regularly see patients who have been referred to me with the diagnosis of pulmonary hypertension. At their first visit, I ask them, "Do you know what pulmonary hypertension is? Has your doctor explained what the implications are, what that diagnosis means for you?"

Two-thirds of the patients have not been informed. They say, "Some kind of high blood pressure" or "I think I have been referred to you so you can prescribe an expensive pulmonary hypertension drug." The other third of the patients Google "pulmonary hypertension," find the Pulmonary Hypertension Association (PHA) website, and read everything they can find on the Internet. They are usually confused and scared.

As I sit down with my newly referred patient and her spouse to provide the information and tell them the truth, I wonder why the referring physician did not take the time to provide some answers.

After information and truth telling follows the informed consent. Enrollment of a patient in any clinical study requires an "informed consent," which begins with the description of the problem. Then there is a discussion of what can be done about the problem—all the options that are known, including the option of doing nothing.

Tom Petty applied this principle when dealing with his severely and chronically ill patients. After he had treated his patients for many years with medications and aggressive pulmonary rehabilitation, he would talk with them about how their lung disease would affect them in the end. By then, the patient had a working knowledge of what is called "the work of breathing," firsthand experience of being short of breath with no relief within the patient's or doctor's reach.

The trust that Tom had built over the years with his patients was now transformed into an "informed consent." The information that the patient needs for decision making is this: acute respiratory fatigue after years of chronic lung disease triggers a predictable chain of events: a 911 call, followed by an ambulance transport to the nearest emergency department. The ER physician uses the ABC approach (antibiotic, bronchodilator, corticosteroids) and a non-invasive mask for breathing support. If these measures are ineffective, the patient is intubated and transported to an intensive care unit for mechanical ventilation. The chronic-lung-disease patient knows all of this. What he does not know is that patients with marginal residual lung function cannot be weaned off the mechanical ventilation, or if they should be able to come off mechanical ventilation, their chance of dying during the ensuing twelve months is between 30 and 50 percent. This conversation always triggered the question: "Dr. Petty, do you think that my lung disease has become *that* bad? And can I decide not to be intubated and ventilated?"

"Yes," Tom would say, "your disease has become that bad. We have tried everything. You have been working with the program, and you can refuse mechanical ventilation."

Following this information came the "consent" part. Tom Petty told the patient that he would enter into the medical record that the patient and he had discussed the ventilator option and that after the next patient visit, the patient would decide formally what his wishes were and that this decision would be clearly laid down in the record. The patient would sign the statement that he had been informed and that he would consent to "no intubation." In those days, of course, the medical records were paper documents, and each volume of the patient's medical record would show in bold letters on the cover the words "Do not intubate!"

Tom Petty had not only pioneered oxygen treatment for chronic lung disease patients and organized pulmonary rehabilitation; he had thought through the whole process of patient care, to the bitter end. He would always open another window of hope for his patients as he told them the truth—all of it. His patients loved him because he understood this "dignity and not losing the control" thing.

So what happens after "Do not intubate"?

There is hospice and home hospice. When the time comes, a nonlethal dose of morphine will numb the respiratory center in the brain and alleviate the air hunger, and a CO_2 (carbon dioxide) narcosis will set in. The fight for the next breath is finally over.

Chapter 12

Comfort Care

All the eighty-five pounds of Suzanne Higgins, lipstick and all, were propped up in her yellow rose of Texas PJs in her bed. She had a double room in the Hospice of St. John, but no roommate. Suzanne had bladder cancer—she once used to smoke a lot when she worked as a realtor in Sun City, Arizona. After her divorce and retirement, she had come to Denver to live with her daughter. The medical director of the hospice was a member of the medical faculty at the university, but it was Father Paul, a descendant from Bohemian nobility and a knight of the order of St. John of Malta, who ran the hospice with an iron fist.[43]

Father Paul had diabetes, and a forefoot amputation made it difficult for him to walk during the last years of his life; however, he was awesomely mobile, courtesy of a high-speed electrical wheelchair that he skillfully steered through the corridors of the ground-level hospice building. Father Paul was loved and feared. The other Paul, the oncologist and medical director of the hospice, told me, "There are only two people I am afraid of: my mother and Father Paul."

After my wife's dad died peacefully from pancreatic cancer in his own bed in his house that he shared with his wife for forty-two years, cared for by a hospice nurse and my mother-in-law, I became interested in hospice care and wanted to know how hospice worked. A few of the medical residents rotated through St. John's, and I tagged along for a few days to see for myself. This is how I met Suzanne and some of the other patients I still remember today.

---

43 Father Paul, actually Prince Paul von Lobkowitz., was a descendant of the Bohemian noble family of von Lobkowitz. They had been highly influential in European political life since the sixteenth century. Beethoven dedicated six string quartets to Franz Joseph von Lobkowitz (1772–1816).

The hospice concept of caring for the dying had been developed over the centuries; for example, the hospice in Beaune in Burgundy, France, financed itself through the sale of wine. But the modern hospice movement was shaped by Dame Cicely Saunders, a British nurse who later became a medical doctor in London. Florence Wald, the Dean of the Yale University School of Nursing, brought the principles of hospice care to America. Since 1971, Hospice Inc. has established hospices all over the United States.

A hospice is run like a hospital, with the exception that life-prolonging—or more to the point, death-delaying treatments—are not administered. Therefore, there is no chemotherapy, no rehab, no bridging to an organ transplant. The idea is to bring end-stage disease to an end—in dignity. Pain treatment is a focus, patients get sleeping pills, and they are fed if they cannot feed themselves. They can have visitors, and there are volunteers who keep patients company, read to them, feed them, and play games with them. On weekends, a volunteer pushes a cart from room to room to deliver alcoholic drinks and ice cream.

Suzanne always had to think about her choice of beverage, but then decided on a highball. Again, this weekend, she had waited for a visit from her daughter, but the daughter had not come. Suzanne tried her best to remain composed and said, "She must have been busy. You know, she works for a big company."

She looked at the tall glass on her nightstand, took a sip, and said: "It is very strong, but not too strong." Then she added, "Look what I did! My lipstick is all over the glass." Her mind wandered off, but then she tried out some small talk.

Smoking was not allowed in the rooms, but patients in wheelchairs, if they wanted to smoke, could do so in the courtyard, which has a fountain, wind chimes, and pretty flowers. In the summer, there are bees and butterflies, and birds visit several feeders.

There were patients with varying degrees of dementia, but there was also a thirty-five-year-old Mexican man with end-stage liver disease. His beer ration was six cans per day, and he was allowed to visit the refrigerator and help himself to a Bud, which he did, like clockwork.

Father Paul was omnipresent and knew who of the patients wanted to just talk or pray with him. The hospice was a rather quiet place and featured an aquarium with goldfish in the entrance hall. All you heard was the muffled sound of television sets, some patients reading newspapers, and occasionally a room door closing. There was a death watch. No patient was supposed to die alone. A nurse was there in the room to hold a patient's hand when there were no relatives. They told me there was usually no fear, no pain—rather a good death.

The Hospice of St. John has a small library containing a few hundred books for those who can still read and turn pages. The last time I saw Suzanne, she was sitting on the edge of her bed. Her skinny legs were dangling from the bed; on a side table on which she could lean, she had a coffee-table-size book of paintings of the French painter Paul Cezanne— landscapes and still-life paintings printed on glossy paper. She did not know anything of the life and career of this painter who had worked in his studio in Aix-en-Provence in the South of France and painted Mt. St. Victoire over and over again until he died in 1905 of pneumonia. She smiled as she looked at the pictures. She closed one eye with one hand and then the other and said, "I like the colors, and the light...." She said the light reminded her of Arizona, where she had lived all of her life. Like most patients at St. John's, Suzanne knew that she was in this place so she could die. At my next visit, her room was empty, but the Cezanne book was still on the table.

As we have recognized the distinction between "futile care" and "palliative care," more patients in the United States nowadays choose hospice care. In 2008, more than 900,000 patients did so. A large amount of the funding for hospice services comes from Medicare.

"Do good and disappear," Father Paul was known to say. "Serve and leave." He had founded the second hospice in America and had served for twenty-seven years. Father Paul died in 2004, a Knight of the Order of St. John, a modern-day crusader fighting for a humane medicine—one patient at a time. One of my heroes.

Chapter 13

Halloween Does Not Do It

It was Dia de Los Muertos (the day of the dead) in Puebla, Mexico. The Mexican Cardiology Society had invited me to give a talk about pulmonary hypertension and heart failure. I had been invited before by the Mexican pulmonary hypertension group to attend the biannual meeting of the society, and this was my third visit to Mexico. Public sites everywhere were decorated. There were shrines at each street corner and shrines and displays covering the city's main square in front of the cathedral. Teenage girls painted each other's faces white and drew deep black rings around the eyes and the mouth. They were the living dead.

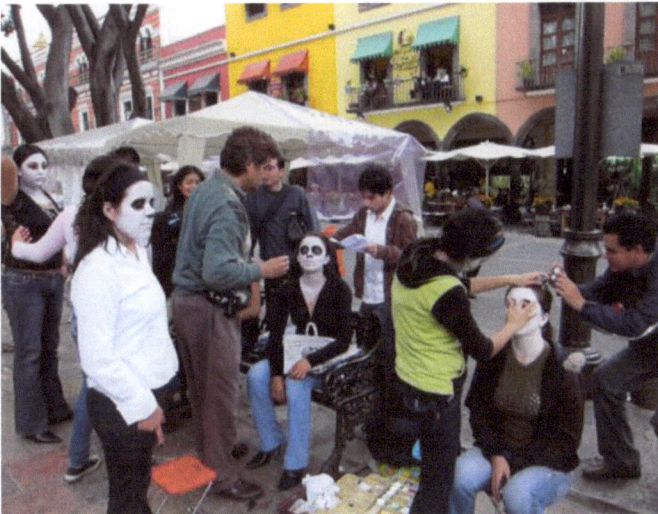

There were dancing and beer-drinking skeletons, skulls made of sugar, and altars adorned with beans and grains. A young woman was dressed as Frida Kahlo, the painter wife of the artist and muralist Diego Rivera. Her eyebrows were painted so they would grow together above her nose, and she smoked a cigar. Role play and impersonation abounded, and the dominant colors were black and orange. Marigolds were everywhere.

The photo shows a street scene in Puebla, Mexico, on the day of the dead. The square in front of the cathedral is packed with people celebrating , wearing masks and building elaborate displays.

While American children are more treating than tricking on the day known as Halloween, in Mexico there is a celebration of the dead; offerings are made (ofrendas), and they consist of packs of cigarettes, if the deceased liked to smoke, or bottles of beer. Parents take pictures of their young children carrying papier-mâché or marigold crosses. Every year on this day, the people remind each other that death is part of life.

After I left Puebla, the following weekend I found myself back on service in the medical intensive care unit and having the following conversation. I was the attending of record (AOR). I got a call from a doctor working in a small county hospital. He wanted to transfer a patient to us. I asked, "What is the problem?"

The doctor replied, "She has kidney failure, and they can't do dialysis."

Hard to believe—there are dialysis units literally everywhere. So I asked, "How old is the patient?"

The doctor on the phone said: "She is ninety-four."

I asked back: "So why do you need to transfer her?"

"Her family wants everything done!"

"Who is the family?" I asked.

"She has a niece! I told the niece that without dialysis, her aunt would die. The niece has the power of attorney."

"Does the patient have a living will?"

"No, there is no living will, and the old lady is not very much with it. She would not understand what 'dialysis' means."

At that time, the chair of the hospital ethics committee (CEC) overheard the conversation and joined in. He is a medical doctor and a lawyer. He is friendly and exuberant and has a sense of humor, but he is the kind of guy who lets you know in a subtle way that he knows and *you* don't.

"We should talk about this. I mean, what's the right thing to do in this case? Hippocrates says just because you are ninety-four does not mean you should die. I think we all agree." The admitting resident listened attentively. He was on call and would have to admit this patient if the transfer were approved by the AOR.

"By the way, is the lady African American?" the CEC asked." No", said the AOR.

Regardless, the CEC started lecturing;"As you know, matters of life and dying should be very carefully avoided—at least initially with these folks. These folks believe that talking about dying puts the kibosh on the patient, and the relatives believe that the patient *will* die. The other point is that we really should not advise the patient too much because this would be paternalistic. The patient remains the decision maker!"

AOR: "But we do not have a living will, and the patient is apparently in no shape to make a decision." The AOR realized that the small-hospital referring physician was still waiting on the phone.

"We have to figure this out. I have only two ICU beds open at the moment. I will call you back," I, the AOR, said and hung up.

Now assured of the undivided attention of his audience, the CEC proposed this: "Get the rest of the team, and let's go to the conference room and examine the matter in a rational fashion." The admitting resident excused himself because he had to admit a patient who had just rolled in—that left one ICU bed.

The CEC said, "Let's look at the dynamics of this situation: Here is the poor country doctor out there who can't handle the kidney failure. Then there is the niece who says that everything has to be done. And there is this ICU with one bed left."

I listened and could not stop thinking, *What about the ninety-four-year-old lady, the patient? Who are we treating? he country doctor? The niece?*

The conversation finally moved to quality of life. The AOR, talking to the referring physician on his iPhone, found out that the patient, prior to her kidney failure, had been essentially bedridden. When he heard this, the CEC said, "This may be a slippery slope. Discussing the best outcome scenario of bedridden plus dialysis three times a week with the doctor may be unwise, particularly if the niece should be a lawyer. It is smarter to say, 'Sorry, we do not have a bed open right now.'" He smiled like a prosecutor who had won his case, leaving the team behind as he sailed through the door. A decision had been made for us.

Perhaps things would be different in this country if we would celebrate Dia de Los Muertos. For the most part, members of the community of health care providers are uncomfortable with the principle of "Just because we *can* do this does not mean that we *should* do this." End-of-life care remains a minefield—and not only an ethical one. Humane conduct collides with market interests. We are dealing with the slippery slope, the reality of litigation, length of hospital stay and survival statistics, and community practice standards. Who is to be the judge? Just because we can do this....

The next day, the CEC returned to the ICU and asked, "Just for my interest, did you guys end up taking that ninety-four- year-old lady?"

Chapter 14

Quality Assessment and Online Reputation Management

As the aging American population is starting to deal with the burden of its diseases, ever better informed about new breakthroughs in stem cell biology and advances in cancer treatment, there are groups and institutions like the Institute for Family Health that are proposing new health care models to address the three key problems that we face: access to care without obstacles, improving quality of health care, and cost reduction. There is a journal published by the American College of Medical Quality ,*American Journal of Medical Quality*, and in this and in other journals, one can read about efforts to link the legislation formulated in the Affordable Care Act, also known as Obamacare, with Accountable Care Organizations (ACOs). ACOs are understood as "affiliations of health care providers that are held jointly accountable for achieving improvements in the quality of care and reductions in spending." Individuals interested in the ACO model can attend workshops and conferences—for a fee—and learn about the "challenges associated with financing, assembling, and developing a quality of care model for successful ACO execution." ACO engineers propose to introduce an "expanded denominator" that would ensure that ACOs are held accountable not only for patients already engaged in primary care, but also for patients with fragmented care and high-risk community members.[44]

And here is another recent statement:

One of the three goals for accountable care organizations is to improve population health. This will require that ACOs bridge the schism between clinical care and public health. But do health care

---

44 N.S. Calman, et al., "Lost to Follow-Up: The public Health Goals of Accountable Care, Arch Intern Med 172, no. 7 (2012) 584-6.

delivery organizations and public health agencies share a concept of "population"? We think not: Whereas delivery systems define populations in term of persons receiving care, public health agencies typically measure health on the basis of geography. This creates an attribution problem, particularly in large urban centers, where multiple health care providers often serve any given neighborhood.[45]

So how can the ACO concept work in a field of competing and attributing stakeholders and shareholders?

Is this one of the problems? Perhaps American health care is over-administered, over-regulated, and altogether too defensive. There appears to be not a problem not only with the assessment of quality issues, but apparently there are also problems with the image of some of the care providers. That is where "reputation management" comes to the rescue.

The website www.reputation.com will make sure that the truth comes out; the company behind the website puts together a plan to promote a physician's areas of expertise and to increase the ranking of positive information about the physician. The website emphasizes research and near-perfect patient scores the physician has received on www.vitals.com and will publish the doctor's pursuits beyond medicine, such as receiving a volunteer award for his work at the local fire station. I was recently contacted by another website, www.healthtap.com. The advertisement stated that because of "glowing articles in the national media, millions of people are looking for your expertise on Health Tap." About this website, *The Wall Street Journal* said this:

> Health Tap enables physicians to market themselves and build their clientele by attracting millions of patients online and through mobile devices, where users are able to see [doctors'] impressive credentials. Health Tap keeps the cyberchondria at bay. Sign up today to get featured in this special Health Tap forum and bring widespread attention to your practice.

---

45 M.N. Gourevitch, et al. "The Challenge of Attributions: Responsibility for Population Health in the Context of Accountable Care," American Journal of Public Health 42, no. 6 (2012) 5180-83.

Late in 2011, the Washington State Health Care Authority announced its intention to stop paying for emergency department visits by Medicaid beneficiaries when these visits are not necessary. A list of non-emergency conditions including acute bronchitis, headache, and urinary tract infection was generated and, presumably, patients with these ailments are turned away or receive a bill after their visit. This is another example of contradicting principles: accountable care—if it is organized—and, on the other hand, access denied by state governments searching for ways out of Medicaid spending.[46] One medical journal said the following:

> Choosing among metrics is as much about values and priorities as about science, and it directly affects health policy.... An ideal, sophisticated health policy would integrate measures of morbidity and the impact that the disease has on people's ability to lead meaningful, productive lives to form a holistic map of the burden of disease[47].

How do we "form this holistic map"? We declare that "perhaps 10 percent of premature deaths are explained by health care as conventionally delivered—when compared with other factors, including social context, environmental influences, and personal behavior." And we postulate that "today's standard approach of reimbursing for office visits and hospitalizations is likely to be displaced once better measures of outcomes can provide a substitute that's more relevant to our key goals. If we can measure success, why pay for process?"[48]

Maybe this is a bit over the top, but you get a feel for the language.

---

46 A.L. Kellermann, et al., "Emergency Departments, Medicaid Costs, and Access to Primary Care—Understanding the Link," New England Journal of Medicine 366, no. 23 (2012) 2141-43.

47 D. Jones, et al., "The Burden of Disease and the Changing Task of Medicine, New England Journal of Medicine 366, no. 25 (2012) 2333-38.

48 D.A. Asch, et al., "What Businesses Are We In? The Emergence of Health as the Business of Health Care," New England Journal of Medicine 367, no. 10 (2012) 888-89.

Chapter 15

Self-Inflicted Injuries

My earliest memory of morbid obesity—I would later call it the "beached whale syndrome"—goes back to the days when I was a pulmonary fellow. I was called to see a patient. The request for consultation was "The patient doesn't breathe." I went to see the patient. There was a 45-year-old woman weighing somewhere around 450 pounds, flat on her back—snoring. Her lips were blue, and indeed, there was only an occasional breath, a gurgling sound of air intake followed by a long pause. She was difficult to wake up, ready to doze off. As I tried to examine her, I found that she could not be moved and that my stethoscope was useless. I could not hear heart sounds; I could not hear breath sounds. I thought that there was probably a pulse. The technical term for this fatal disorder is obesity/hypoventilation syndrome, and we do not fully understand how patients get to this state of morbid obesity.

Charles Dickens introduced the literary protagonist of this disease, "Fat Joe," in his first novel, *The Posthumous Papers of the Pickwick Club*, also known as the "Pickwick Papers." Fat Joe would fall asleep on his carriage, the reigns of his team of horses dropping out of his hands, until the bumping up and down in his carriage on the cobblestone streets of London woke him up. In short, the problem of this woman was morbid obesity aggravated by respiratory failure. These patients have a penchant for hiding in their homes for many years, avoiding most or all social contact until someone finds them ready to die—and then they are hospitalized. For some years, I have argued with my endocrinologist friends that this disease could not simply be the consequence of overeating. I was searching for genetic reasons and decided on a hypothesis of a systems biology disorder. Understanding diseases in terms of system biology de-emphasizes the one-organ-disease locus. The theory rather calls for a concept of integrated systems failure, as, for example, captured by the term "neuroendocrine immune disorder."

This is a mouthful, but the term conveys that three systems are jointly in disarray: the brain, the endocrine system, and the immune system. When it comes to morbid obesity, unfortunately now predicted to become the fate of millions of American children, the use of this term opens up the view toward a failure of the brain/endocrine axis, which also affects normal immune system functions.

Contemplating potential genetic determinants of this syndrome, as a pulmonary fellow, I had no particular insights or knowledge of the genetics of obesity, but I remember my shock and disbelief when I recognized that, shortly after my failed attempts to examine the patient, two more 350-pounders had entered the room—the unfortunate woman's daughters.

Maybe I am off here, but I continue to believe that this obesity epidemic that is now upon us in America is not completely explainable by the combination of overeating and lack of exercise. Some of the consequences and downstream effects of obesity are now explained by "inflammation." In essence, inflammatory cells contained in the fat pad release factors that circulate and affect other organs, and some of these factors are powerful angiogenic (they generate new blood vessels) molecules; capillaries must grow so that the fat pad can grow.

The genetic component is being investigated to some degree in the studies of the Pima Indians in Arizona. On one of my trips to the Grand Canyon, I discovered a side canyon where the Havasupai tribe lives. The Havasupai people have been living there for more than a thousand years and were sheltered from civilization until recently. A modest tourist industry has changed this now; the Havasupais have been discovered by hikers and Sierra Club members. The Indian settlements are spread around the banks of the Colorado River and were once difficult to get to. Now, one can drive to a parking lot and trailhead about ten miles from the canyon bottom, strap a backpack on, and hike down a winding donkey trial through trees and rocks. As you move slowly down the trail, it does not escape your attention that both sides of the trail are littered with cans that were once filled with soda drinks: Pepsi, Mountain Dew, Dr Pepper, Fanta, Orange Crush—you name it. The Indians transport the cans on pack horses and mules, and they make two daily trips to the parking lot and back. As you hike down and come to the end of the trail, you find a little village at the bottom of the canyon, a trading post, and an air-conditioned restaurant—and there you

92

instantaneously get it: The people are all big. The men, women, boys, and girls are all supersized, and many have one of these soda cans in their hand. It turns out that many of the people living around the beautiful emerald pools at the canyon bottom drink four to six cans of their favorite beverage a day (140 calories x 6) of a mixture of corn sugar, taste bud teasers, and food dyes. The hypothesis is that the native Indians are genetically unprepared for the overdose of carbohydrates that they now have easy access to in the form of the macaroni and cheese dinners, the pizzas, and the rest of the processed and colorfully packed foods they find in the supermarkets. The Indians had, for hundreds of years, survived on a subsistence diet of beans, nuts, and fish and the occasional deer and elk. Corn in the Rio Grande basin was and is a sacred plant that was planted and harvested ritually. "Corn mothers" were piled on shrines in the houses or in caves, and the mischievous Kokopelli guarded the corn fields. Corn meant bread, and there was never enough of it.

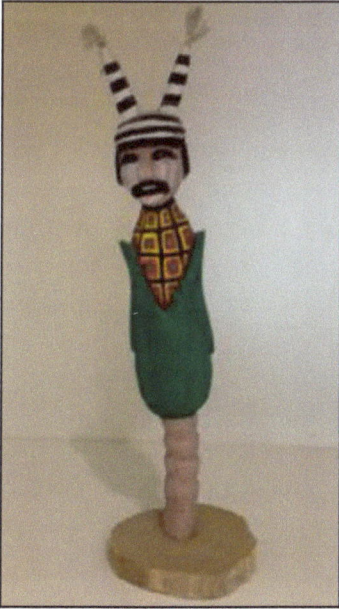

This Hopi kachina cotton wood sculpture shows a koshare (a trickster/ruffian, who makes his appearance during the ceremonial dances of the southwestern pueblo Indians, and a member of the "two horn" society) emerging from a corn plant. This is an interesting iconic depiction /fusion of fertility and creativity.

Now the highly genetically conserved descendants of these original Rio Grande tribes take in gallons of corn syrup in addition to cookies and breakfast bars that are also laced with corn syrup. The Arizona-based nonprofit organization Native Seeds/SEARCH now distributes Tepary beans to Indian tribes in the Southwest. The beans don't need much water to grow and are low in carbohydrates.

So the starting point for the obesity problem—soon to be a national disaster—is hypothetically the toxic corn sugar (fructose) calorie load that, together with a required genetic disposition in these individuals, and soon patients—is preferentially metabolized to fat.

Perhaps, and I am wildly speculating, our intestinal bacterial flora (the gut biotome) gets "drunk" on corn sugar, a bacterial selection occurs as a consequence, and the altered gut flora adversely affect intestinal foodstuff absorption and the way carbohydrates are metabolized.

This hypothesis may be wrong but should be investigated. Even if only "somewhat" true, then one would have to see morbid obesity not strictly as a self-inflicted disease, but as a combination of genetics and a malignant environment—i.e., toxic sugars. If so, then the image of the obese patient sitting on her porch sipping her Dr Pepper provides at least two of the clues to the problem.

Obesity is an enormous health problem. More and more children and adolescents are now overweight or obese. Obesity comes with diabetes, asthma, and sleep apnea and an increased cancer risk. A cross-sectional survey of 4,456 participants representing 195 million adults aged 20–79 years in the 2003–2004 National Health and Nutrition Examination Survey (NHANES) found abdominal obesity to be present in 42 percent of men and 62 percent of women.[49] Experts continue to discuss whether obesity is a behavioral or endocrine disorder.

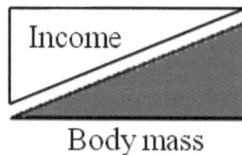

Body mass

In the United States, 16.9 percent of children and adolescents aged 2–19 years are now obese.[50] There is apparently a strong relationship between

49 E. Ghandehari, et al., "Abdominal Obesity and the Spectrum of Global Cardiometabolic Risks in US Adults," Int. J. Obesity 33, no. 2 (2009) 239-48.
50 C.L. Ogden, et al., "Prevalence in High Body Mass Index in US Children and Adolescents, 2007–2008," Journal of the American Medical Association 307 no. 5 (2010)

household income and body weight. Only 18 percent of Americans consider external factors like exposure to junk food and a limited availability to healthy food as the biggest causes of childhood obesity, while 64 percent identify overeating, lack of exercise, and watching too much television as the biggest causes.[51]

The doctor can prescribe lifestyle changes, but the patient must lose the weight. Every decade or so, the pharmaceutical industry markets weight-loss pills. These prescription drugs come with warning labels. The so-called Fen/Phen combination caused heart valve problems and pulmonary hypertension—in many cases with a lethal outcome, as already mentioned. The arguments made by proponents of weight-loss drugs and their prescribers are that the patients can't lose weight, they need help, and any amount of weight loss that can be induced is beneficial. This argument is seriously flawed simply because most obese people, after stopping the diet pills, gain their weight right back!

I still remember the large billboards advertising the services of law firms: "If you have had a problem related to Fen/Phen, call us." Physicians had used the same billboards ten years earlier. Their ads had read, "If you want to lose weight, we have Fen/Phen. Give us a call!"

For a few years, I provided expertise for lawyers who represented patients (plaintiffs) who had developed severe pulmonary hypertension after they had been treated with the appetite suppressant fenfluramine. I was deposed by lawyers representing the drug company. The first deposition stretched over two days, six hours each day, and I quickly realized that my assessments of the relationship of drug intake and pulmonary hypertension and my concepts of the cause of pulmonary hypertension became part of the public record. Other lawyers would, in later depositions, make every effort to provoke statements that would contradict my opinions and statements that I had uttered during this first deposition. One of the lawyers who deposed me wore a Jaws t-shirt—yes, the widely exposed dentistry of a great white shark; another lawyer wore a "Where's Waldo?" tie; for a few hours, I searched for Waldo.

483-90.
51 C.L. Barry, S.E. Gollust, and J. Niederdeppe, "Are Americans Ready to Solve the Weight of the Nation?" *New England Journal of Medicine* 367, no. 5 (2012) 389-91.

We still do not really understand how fenfluramine causes pulmonary hypertension in genetically susceptible people. And that is, in large part, due to the fact that we do not have an animal model. Apparently drug-induced pulmonary hypertension requires genes that are expressed only in humans. Feeding these appetite-suppressing drugs to mice or rats does not cause pulmonary hypertension. This means that there is really no way to screen for drug-induced pulmonary hypertension.

The market demands diet pills. Two new drugs were released in the summer of 2012. Will we have to face drug-induced pulmonary hypertension again?

Chapter 16

It's What You Need to Know, Not What You Want to Know

There are thousands of Long Term Acute Care (LTAC) hospitals in America. These facilities accept patients after they have been discharged from a regular acute care hospital, usually too sick to return to their home or to a nursing home. Many patients in these fully staffed hospitals require chronic ventilator care. Regular large-city hospitals and the university health sciences centers with their emergency departments, outpatient clinics, and intensive care medicine units nowadays keep more patients alive than they can house. Whereas the intake of patients occurs mainly through the emergency department or direct admissions for scheduled procedures and surgery, the outtake or discharge of patients who are not well enough to function independently after they have survived a life-threatening illness has become problematic. The beds are needed for the new patients waiting at the gates.

LTACs emerged about thirty years ago, designed to provide an environment for the weaning of ventilator-dependent patients. LTAC hospitals are now part of the health care industry, with for-profit corporations dominating the field. One large conglomerate charts annual revenue of $6 billion, generated by more than 76,000 employees in forty-six US states. Medicare recognizes 432 LTAC hospitals.[52]

About 10 to 20 percent of patients recovering from a critical illness require long-term specialized care for a prolonged period of time. Kahn, et al., assessed that admissions increased from 50.7 percent in 2000 to 52.2 percent in 2006. About 40 percent of the patients who required ventilation at the LTAC facility survived 100 days. David Scheinhorn and his

---

52 J.M. Kahn, et al., "Long-Term Acute Care Hospitals Utilization after Critical Illness, Journal of the American Medical Association 303, no. 22 (2010) 2253-59.

colleagues examined 1,419 patients in twenty-three LTAC hospitals and found that the median age of the patients was seventy-two years. A medical illness led to ventilator dependency in 61 percent of the cases, and a surgical procedure led to ventilator dependency in 39 percent of the patients. More than 80 percent have at least three penetrating indwelling tubes or catheters[53]

We need to remind ourselves that 5 percent of the American patients account for about 50 percent of the American health care costs. Who are these 5 percent? They are the patients with end-stage chronic diseases and end-stage cancer and patients in the intensive care units. Treatment strategies that are futile and prolong dying account for some of these costs. Today we should be able to assess the morbidities and co-morbidities that determine a bad outcome following major surgical procedures and advise patients and their families not to have these risky procedures. It is important for Boomers to know these statistics, and they need to have advanced directives written down! They need to document what their intentions and wishes are in case they have a chronic or life-threatening illness.

---

53 Scheinhorn, DJ et al. Ventilator-dependent survivors of catastrophic illness transferred to 23 long-term care hospitals for weaning from prolonged mechanical ventilation. Chest, 131, no. 1 (2007 76-84).

Chapter 17

Public and Not-So-Public Debates about Health Care

In the 2012 election year, starting with the Republican primaries and continuing after the elections, health care policies, legislation, and budget-deficit-driving health care costs were a topic for morning talk shows and television attack advertisements. On June 29th, a Thursday, the US Supreme Court ruled that the key components of the Affordable Care Act would stand, and it appears that the legislation will be implemented in 2014. It was a 5:4 decision, and most commentators professed amazement that Chief Justice John Roberts joined the less conservative wing of the court. By the weekend, analysts had their sources explain that the Chief Justice had originally decided to vote against the ACA, or large parts of it, and then later changed his mind (for political reasons?) and sided with the minority. It was newsworthy.

When did he do it? Why did he do it? Thereafter, the conversations were about the mandate to buy health insurance, whether citizens could be forced to buy insurance, and whether or not failing to buy insurance would result in a penalty or a tax. While experts and commentators had a field day, hospital companies were looking at a windfall because the ACA will provide coverage for several millions of previously uninsured. As Texas state legislator Debbie Riddle once said so succinctly, "Where did this idea come from that everybody deserves free education, free medical care, free whatever? It comes from Moscow, from Russia. It comes straight out of the pit of hell." Here you have it—a functional health care system would be hell.

And the governor of the great state of Louisiana was heard saying, "That's why we need to vote for Mitt Romney, because he will destroy 'Obamacare.'"

Torrents of anger flow through the landscape of American health care. The bare-knuckle all and out fight for control of the agenda will not settle anything but surely will confuse millions of citizens, and actions taken to dismantle the ACA legislation may have devastating consequences—at least in the short run. In the end, what will replace the destroyed Obamacare, which really is a variation of Romneycare?

There is one fact on which we have great clarity: While the expansion of Medicaid in the states that will participate and accept the federal dollars will provide access to the health care system for many people, the ACA will still leave eleven million undocumented people without coverage and will likely make it more difficult for the undocumented to gain access to basic primary care services. For some, the Affordable Care Act has become the affordable "scare" act.

What is frighteningly apparent is the lack of concepts regarding the root causes of the dilemma and the absence of a real reform idea. Nobody says publicly, "We must rebuild American health care from the ground up." Nobody wants to acknowledge that the healing arts need to be protected from the greed of Wall Street. If the American health care industry—like the banking industry in 2008—were to hit rock bottom next year, there is no vision (nothing I can find) of how to build a better system. None of the politicians have studied other systems or programs well enough to recommend alternatives. Most American physicians find it a waste of time to study health care systems in other countries. As we heard already from Texas, the boogie man is socialism. Yet social Darwinism is acceptable.

Then there are those people who are shouting, "I am tired of paying for everybody else's stupidities" and "Why do I have to pay for the smokers and overeating couch potatoes?" Sandeep Jauhar wrote the following on March 29, 2010 under the headline :No Matter What, We Pay for Others Bad Habits in *The New York Times*:

"Personal responsibility is a complex notion, especially when it comes to health. Individual choices always take place within a broader, messy context. When people advocate the need for personal accountability, they presuppose more control over health and sickness than really exists.... Unhealthy habits are certainly one factor, but so are social status, income, family dynamics, education, and genetics.

100

The problem is that punitive measures to force healthy behavior do not usually work. In 2006, West Virginia started rewarding Medicaid patients who signed a pledge to enroll in a wellness plan and to follow their doctor's orders with special benefits, including unlimited prescription drug coverage, programs to help them quit smoking, and nutrition counseling. The program, by many accounts, is failing. As of August 2009, only 15 percent of 160,000 eligible patients had signed up. Patients with limited transportation options had had a hard time committing to regular office visits. And experts say that there is no evidence that restricting benefits for noncompliant patients has promoted healthy behaviors."

Yes, but there is the mayor of New York City, Michael Bloomberg. First he banned smoking in restaurants. The European Respiratory Society gave him an award, and he flew to Berlin to receive the award at its conference. It has been estimated that New York City's anti-smoking measures, which also included an increased tobacco tax, decreased the smoking population by 450,000 over a decade and the number of smoking-related deaths by nearly 1,500. Bloomberg moved on to trans fats, and recently he started the "soda wars." New York City plans to ban the sale of supersized sugary drinks—no more super Slurpees. Of course you can buy three or four regular-size drinks. Notably, the spokesman of the New York City Beverage Association countered, "The New York City health department's unhealthy obsession with attacking soft drinks.... It's time for serious health professionals to move on and seek solutions that are actually going to cure obesity."[54] Tell that to the Havasupai or Pima Indians in Arizona.

Three new studies, recently published, provide data showing that the consumption of sugar-sweetened beverages may influence the development of obesity in children. A study by Qi, et al., provides strong evidence for an interaction between intake of sugar-sweetened beverages and a genetic obesity predisposition.[55]

---

54 M.M. Grynbaum, The New York Times, New York Plans to Ban Sale of Big Sizes of Sugary Drinks May 30, 2012.
55 S. Caprio, "Calories from Soft Drinks—Do They Matter?" New England Journal of Medicine 367, no. 15 (2012) 1462-63.

Sonia Caprio writes in the *New England Journal of Medicine*: "Sugar intake from sugar-sweetened beverages alone, which are the largest single caloric food source in the United States, approaches 15 percent of the daily caloric intake in several population groups. Adolescent boys in the United States consume an average of 357 kcal of the beverages per day. Large increases in consumption of sugar-sweetened beverages have occurred among black and Mexican-American youth, who are known to be at higher risk for obesity and the development of type II diabetes than their counterparts."[56] As mentioned before, sugar-sweetened drinks contain fructose from corn syrup. High-fructose corn syrup has been shown to increase blood pressure.[57] Some investigators are still holding out, stating that the evidence for high-fructose corn syrup causing an increase in visceral fat deposition is still inconclusive. That reminds me of the days when the tobacco industry ran advertisements stating, "Your doctor smokes Chesterfield."

Recently, journalist Fareed Zakaria said on CNN, "American health care is a mess." I agree.

---

56 G. Block, "Foods Contributing to Energy Intake in the US: Data from NHANES III and NHANES 1999–2000," J. Food Comp Anal. 17, no. 3-4 (2004) 439-47.

57 M.T. Le, et al., "Effects of High-Fructose Corn Syrup and Sucrose on the Pharmacokinectics and Acute Metabolic and Hemodynamic Responses in Healthy Subjects," Metabolism 61, no. 5 (2012) 641-51.

Chapter 18

The Mystical Wisdom of the Market

For some time now, I have been looking for the "invisible hand" that guides the American health care market. I have listened to the morning news driving to the hospital, stuck in traffic watching the windshield wipers moving the heavy downpour, as the commentator announces the following:

> Since two-thousand-two, during the last decade, the mortality from heart attacks has decreased by forty-six percent. How did this happen? We have looked at the entire system from the first-call emergency response team to the coronary intervention in the hospital. The emergency medical technicians (EMTs) are all well trained. The system works. The EMTs get to the patient with chest pain after the nine-one-one call in a flash, the patient chews an aspirin tablet, and if the electrocardiogram shows that there is a serious ischemic problem with the heart, a pattern consistent with a fresh, evolving infarct, then the patient is driven to a hospital that has an interventional cardiology service. The emergency room physician is notified and the cardiology team as well. The goal is to have the patient in the heart catheterization lab on the table within ninety minutes after onset of the chest pain.

The spokesperson for the Health Department continues to explain the principle of early intervention—to reopen the blocked artery as soon as possible and to salvage the threatened and otherwise dying heart muscle. She explains that the awareness campaign of the American Heart Association, the training of more and more citizens in basic cardiac life support techniques, and the use of defibrillators have had an impact on survival after a cardiac arrest. Indeed, easy-to-use defibrillators that signal whether there is a "shockable" heart rhythm have spread and can be found in most American airports. They also are stored in the medicine cabinets of all airplanes.

Sudden death can occur without coronary artery disease due to catastrophic heart rhythm disturbances. If such an event strikes a young athlete on the soccer field or basketball court and is recorded by television cameras, then the story makes the evening news. The sudden death of a national soccer team player in Spain had recent consequences. The Minister of Health ordered that all professional athletes needed to have an extensive cardiac exam, including an echocardiogram (a cardiac ultrasound study that provides images of the cardiac chambers and the cardiac valves in motion), something like an "engine check." Tens of thousands of athletes were checked, and a new medicine market segment had been discovered.

By far, the worst outcome after a successful cardiac resuscitation is brain death—no cardiac pump action, no blood flow to the brain. Although a long, so-called down time makes recovery of brain function unlikely, there are too many factors involved to make accurate predictions. Rapid cooling of the circulating blood (hypothermia) following a cardiac arrest and return of the pump function is a strategy that is now employed in a number of heart centers in America, and full recovery of the patient post-cardiac arrest is no longer rare and anecdotal[58] "Shock, cool, and save a brain" requires a large and well-trained team of first responders and specialists with expertise in hibernation and thermoregulation. Perhaps we are at the threshold of a new era of medicine, which I will name cryotherapy.

Of course it is all about energy, about slowing down the metabolism. It is also about machines. Our modern medical care undoubtedly has been advanced by modern electronics, machines, support systems, and expensive equipment. We make use of membrane oxygenators and dialysis machines, and we implant pacemakers and defibrillators. Plus, there are balloon pumps and left ventricular assist devices (artificial hearts), small programmable pumps for the infusion of insulin and delivery of drugs that lower the blood pressure. We insert drug-coated stents into coronary arteries, we ultrasound the bronchial tree, and we engineer cells.

---

58 A.C. Heffner, et al., "Regionalization of Post-Cardiac Arrest Care: Implementation of a Cardiac Resuscitation Center," *American Heart Journal* 164, no. 4 (2012) 493–501 e2.

There are now centers in Texas specializing in stem cell therapy. A lump of abdominal fat is removed. Then cells are isolated, sorted, and expanded in culture for several weeks and injected into the patient's vein, costing $7,000 for two hundred thousand cells. This procedure is repeated two to three times. Does the cell therapy work? Nobody knows.

The spectrum of diagnostic and therapeutic options is expanding rapidly. We have biologicals: antibodies, growth factors, and cells from an umbilical cord. We can transplant kidneys, hearts, livers, lungs, skin, retinas, pancreas cells, and bone marrow. We remove "bad humors" from the blood via plasmapheresis and replace faulty proteins like alpha1antitrypsin in patients with the genetic defect that leads to abnormal folding of this protein and emphysematous destruction of their lungs. Patients born with another hereditary disease, hemophilia (lack of a coagulation factor causes bleeding), survive on substitution of this factor, and patients with sickle cell anemia regularly receive blood exchange transfusions.

Entrepreneurial health care engineers have many ideas. Some advocate that every child's umbilical cord blood, which is rich in stem cells, should be frozen and saved for a repair of destroyed or malfunctioning organs later in life. There is the implantable microchip containing your entire health care record—computed tomography (CT) images included—as well as your entire genome. There are dozens of applications (apps) for your cell phone that allow you to calculate your daily caloric intake and to input your daily weight, blood sugar values, blood pressure numbers, and the distance you walk in twenty-four hours. The phone reminds you to take your medicine and to reorder your medications, and it automatically sounds an alarm the moment you approach a McDonald's restaurant.

This body of yours generates energy, burns energy. The heart muscle has a very high energy requirement. The energy units of living organisms are ATP (the small adenosine triphosphate), and muscles are fueled by ATP. The heart muscle is interesting because it stores very little ATP energy; it turns over its entire ATP energy resource pool every ten seconds, which amounts to 6 kg of ATP recycled by the adult heart every day.[59] The ATP is generated in the cells by the mitochondrial power plants. A blockage of a

---

59 S. Neubauer, "The Failing Heart—An Engine Out of Fuel," *New England Journal of Medicine* 356, no. 11 (2007) 1140-51.

large coronary artery causes the decrease in available oxygen—as a result of stopped blood flow—in the heart muscle. The archaic mitochondrial power plants know how to switch to alternative energy sources, and some of the heart cells go into hibernation mode to consume less energy. How the heart muscle knows how to switch some, but not all, of the muscle cells to hibernation is still unclear, and research continues in an effort to understand better the structure and function of the tiny mitochondria. Part of the secret of life is hidden in these organelles that make their own DNA and fuse together or replicate within a cell. During a heart attack caused by a critical decrease of heart muscle mitochondria burnout, cells die. Cryotherapy slows down energy consumption and may help mitochondria recover and cells to regain function. Heart function means about one hundred thousand heartbeats a day and the pumping of hundreds of tons of blood per day—much more when we exercise. Normal cells and body function is governed by the principle of energy supply and demand, and it appears that the health care marketplace is driven by demand and limited supplies. In this context, health policy discussions conducted by health care analysts seem to miss the mark and proceed in a vacuum, although well-intentioned. For example, consider this excerpt from a 2012 medical journal article:

> So far, assessment of quality of care and health outcomes has not incorporated patient-centeredness. Outcome measurements have focused on survival and overall mortality. An alternative approach to providing better care would be to focus on a patient's individual health goals within and across a variety of dimensions: symptoms, functional status, social and role functions.... Thus, patients can be in control when treatment options require trade-offs.... Rather than asking what patients want, the culture has valued managing each disease according to guidelines"[59]—and management plans.

What will the health care markets say? Is *this* precision medicine? While some health care analysts discuss "precision medicine," the wisdom of the market is also expressed in statements like these:

"Quality of care is becoming increasingly linked with how physicians are compensated for delivering services. The metrics used to evaluate the quality of care differ depending on the system and change on an almost daily basis."

MD News, a Business Practice Management Magazine[60]

"The National Health Insurer Report Card reveals another lackluster showing from insurers whose claims-processing error rate has risen to nearly 20 percent—resulting in billions of wasted dollars for the health care industry.... Find out how coding discrepancies delayed service, unpaid claims, and other insurance company shortfalls are hitting your practice bottom line."

MD News

Perhaps the healthcare market has no wisdom at all; maybe it is not guided by the supply-and-demand principle. How the energy is generated by health care providers and used by consumer/patients is not a concern. Maybe it's all about "cap and trade" and wasted dollars.... The market's role, its functions?

In some places in the country, the market, the system, has not been hibernating. Hospitals have bought several practices in town—they have consolidated and acquired a greater segment of the market. After that, the rules and conditions of the business can be controlled to decide what tests to run, which patients to admit to the hospital, and how much to charge for procedures and tests.[61]

---

60 D.B. Reuben and M.E. Tinetti, "Goal-Oriented Patient Care—An Alternative Health Outcomes Paradigm," New England Journal of Medicine, 366, no. 9 (2012) 777-79.
61 MD News. Several local editions of this magazine are regularly published by 'True North Custom Media'

Chapter 19

Crafty Intuition, Slim Evidence, and Strong Convictions

It is true—many lawmakers do not want to talk about Medicare and the "mechanics" of the Affordable Care Act. Many appear to be deeply conflicted and talk about American health care only in apocalyptic terms. As most physicians remain silent and just sit and listen, researchers move forward with ingenuity, using ever-shrinking resources. The previous essays have dealt with some of these aspects. Here I want to begin, finally, to highlight some of the strengths of our health care system: the science.

I want to start by quoting the late Solbert Permutt, another pulmonologist, a contemporary of John Murray, and an eminent scholar of lung physiology. A few years back, an old friend from the days in the Cardiovascular Pulmonary Research (CVP) lab, Wiltz Wagner, invited all the living lung researchers who had worked at least twenty-five years in the field of lung circulation (that was his criterion for allowing participation at the meeting) to a conference that was held at the Lost Valley dude ranch in the Colorado Mountains. To this day, I continue to be grateful to Wiltz for having the idea for such a conference and organizing it. All the grey-haired pioneers came and told us "how it really was," how they had asked the fundamental questions of lung biology and then set out to do the research and find the answers. There is, for example, the principle of ventilation/perfusion matching, which is important for the understanding of oxygenation problems in pneumonia and chronic lung diseases. Every medical student is taught this important aspect of lung physiology and struggles to understand how the oxygen level of the circulating blood is regulated by a control mechanism that is unique to the lung. At this "history of lung circulation research" conference, Sol Permutt explained how he had discovered the relationships between air flow and blood flow. He was convinced that the lung blood flow was controlled and not passive—and he had an intuition. He imagined that the blood flow through the lung resembled a waterfall. There are two pipelines in the lung: air pipes and blood pipes. Sol designed experiments in which he could change the pressure in the air compartment and observe how this maneuver would influence the blood flowing in and out of the lung vessels. He also was able to change the amount of blood flowing through the lung arteries, and he could measure how this affected the blood-flow behavior in the veins of the lungs. It was pioneering lung physiology. Add to this the principle of "what part of the lung tissue is not ventilated—shall not be perfused" (because blood flowing through an unventilated part of the lung would not pick up any oxygen and, as a consequence, the body's oxygen concentration would drop) and you have some understanding of this mechanism of ventilation to perfusion matching. Intuition and strong conviction lead to experimental evidence. Permutt's work was later popularized and amended by others, but it is not for that reason that he said this:

> While science is perhaps the most cooperative of all endeavors…it is also confrontational. We thrust and parry ideas like sabers, and we both receive and inflict wounds…. Our papers are rejected, and our grants go unfunded…. The work is hard…but it is a noble battle that we are engaged in, for we fight for the best in science and medicine. We are in the right war at the right time….[62]

Research, a noble battle….

Indeed, medical research and biotechnology in America are the strong backbone of American health care. The war against cancer continues to be fought, and the battle over obesity has been joined. The battlefields are labs in academic institutions and private-sector research labs in thousands of companies that have invested in R & D (research and development). These institutions have assembled research teams (research is a team sport!) that are built on the "critical mass of investigators" principle. The more varied the background knowledge and skill set of the members of the group, the

---

62 R.G. Brower and J.T. Sylvester, "Solbert Permutt, MD, March 6, 1925–May 23, 2012," *American Journal of Respiratory Critical Care Medicine*, 186 (2012) 115.

greater the probability of innovation. Young scientists are attracted to a particular lab because that's where the action is—meaning the new ideas, the excitement of new discoveries, the opportunity to publish in top-tier journals. However, as funding for research is more and more restricted, the National Institutes of Health, one of the command and control centers of US research, insists more and more on the translational potential of the research and is interested in the research product. That is a philosophy not very different from that held by the pharmaceutical industry. The question has become this: At the end of the day, given the best-case scenario, how is your research going to change the diagnosis and treatment of the disease under investigation? Fair enough.

As such, the research community and their proposals are under enormous pressure to identify the most promising pathways that lead from project to product. The product may be a new drug or study results that provide evidence that smoking cigarettes or imbibing high-fructose corn syrup drinks is dangerous for your health.

Perhaps the best-organized and most advanced medical research area is that of cancer research. In 1971, the US Congress expanded the first disease-oriented agency of the NIH, the National Cancer Institute, by passing the National Cancer Act, which created the mandate "to support research and the application of the results of research to reduce the incidence, morbidity, and mortality from cancer." As Vincent DeVita MD, one of the founding fathers of modern cancer chemotherapy, reminisced, "The act would quintuple the budget of the National Cancer Institute by the end of the decade and provide the fuel for the revolution in molecular biology."[63] The mandate of "application of the results" led to the establishment of systematic clinical chemotherapy trials and trials that evaluated the combination of radiation plus chemotherapy or chemotherapy plus surgery. In the late 1960s, the five-year survival of all cancer patients was 38 percent; in 2012, the five-year survival was 68 percent. The breast cancer mortality began to fall in 1991, and we saw the first decrease in the total number of deaths from cancer in 2005.

---

63 V.T. DeVita and S.A. Rosenberg, "Two Hundred Years of Cancer Research," New England Journal of Medicine 366, no. 23 (2012) 2207-14.

As mentioned before, cell- or-tissue-gene expression analysis now can be applied to map the landscape of specific cancers—for example, breast cancer—to identify patients with a low risk of tumor recurrence and those who are resistant or susceptible to different forms of chemotherapy. (Oncologist Dr. Lukas Wartman had his leukemia cells genotyped). It is expected that our knowledge of tumor biology and of driver genes will continue to grow exponentially—i.e., double every five years. New cancer treatments are being developed, and it has been shown that chemoprevention works. In 1998, tamoxifen was found to reduce the incidence of breast cancer, and in 2003, aspirin was found to prevent colon cancer. In 2000, The FDA approved human papilloma virus vaccination for the prevention of uterine cancer.

Some of the academic research centers and teaching hospitals—which provide nearly 40 percent of the country's free care for the 50.7 million uninsured people—fear that the Affordable Care Act will cut payments to hospitals. However, provisions of the law include the Cures Acceleration Network, a NIH grants program aimed at moving drugs and devices into the clinic that the industry has little incentive to develop. There is also the Patient Centered Outcomes Research Institute, which awards grants for research comparing the effectiveness of various treatments.

These are all very positive developments. It is important to find out which treatments work, based on strong evidence, and it is important to find new treatments for crippling autoimmune diseases like lupus and scleroderma and to prevent preventable diseases.

There are other positive developments, too.

Cell biology is making rapid progress in the area of stem cell research. Stem cells were first postulated to exist at the end of the nineteenth century to explain the ability of certain tissues (like blood—yes, blood is a tissue) to self-renew for the lifetime of the organism. Classical experiments had shown that bone marrow, when transplanted to sites in the body that were far away from the bones, would generate at these sites' marrow cells and bone.

There are all sorts of stem cells. Some travel through the blood; others live in niches as resident stem cells in the blood vessels, and still others live in all organs of the body, including the heart. There are embryonic stem cells, cancer stem cells, and the much-talked-about inducible pluripotent stem cells (iPSs). In 2006, two researchers showed, for the first time, that adult mouse cells in the cell culture dish could be reprogrammed and turned into stem cells.[64] Dr. Yamanaka, who had started his career as an orthopedic surgeon, was awarded the 2012 Nobel Prize in Medicine for his discovery of these inducible stem cells.

These paradigm-shifting studies have accelerated stem cell research. Since then, our concepts of how tissues respond to injury and repair themselves—for example, after pneumonia—and of how cancers grow, plus our knowledge of cancer biology, have been greatly influenced. We now have to accept that one normal cell can change into another, different, normal cell. For example, it has been shown that connective tissue cells can be programmed to turn into heart muscle cells and that cells that line blood vessels can be turned into fat cells. Applying the rules and regulations of stem cell biology will be necessary to understand a number of degenerative diseases from heart failure to atherosclerosis and even pulmonary hypertension. After embryonic stem cell research became a political football, now a number of reprogramming methods have been developed to derive these iPSs. Nerve cells, liver cells, skin cells, fat cells, and cartilage cells all have been made, and the question for the bioengineers becomes whether a patient's own cells (for example, skin cells) can be turned into a repair cell to be used to replace or compensate for failing organ cells—for example heart-muscle cells in end-stage heart failure. Instead of bridging patients with terminal heart failure to heart transplantation using artificial mechanical hearts, researchers envision stem cell therapy. Others want to rebuild failing livers and lungs and injured spinal cords. Conceptually, a cell-based therapy would make some of the machines obsolete—comparable to the polio vaccine, which decreased the need for crutches, wheelchairs, and iron lungs. Some people may be frightened by these developments, and cartoonists have a field day depicting shape shifters and multiheaded monsters. Indeed, if this cell reprogramming technology can be applied clinically, much more about the nature and possible fate of engineered cells needs to be known. We don't want bone or fat cells to grow in a failing heart.

---

64 K. Takahashi and S. Yamanaka, "Induction of Pluripotent Stem Cells from Mouse Embryonic and Adult Fibroblast Cultures by DefinedFactors," *Cell* 126, no. 4 (2006) 663-76.

Exciting research is going on in thousands of laboratories in this country. This is very positive. The results of this research can have a great impact, and perhaps soon. Would it not be desirable if some of this energy that drives the biomedical research could be channeled into health care reform?

Chapter 20

Equitable Allocation of Finite Services

The issue that American medicine has become too expensive has been raised again and again on previous pages, and I have attempted to put rising costs and profit optimization into the context of industrialized medicine. Some patients die in intensive care units for too long; defensive medicine is another factor. The corporization of medical services and managed care since 1980 has led to new layers of corporate middle men who increase costs in the name of saving them. Examples could be the army of insurance agents and health benefits managers, as well as the bill-collecting companies, that do not exist in most countries with universal health care.

In a 1976 appraisal of medical education, Rosemary Stevens , a health care historian wrote the following:[65]

> Some may take the view that American medical education is based on the best Europe had to offer: a kind of homespun amalgamation of excellence. From a scientific standpoint that may be true, but besides any such consideration, American medicine in its formative period was based on an essentially practical, no-nonsense approach, which has been submerged, but I hope not lost.... Leading American physicians...were quite clear that common sense was at least as important as science, judgment as learning, and restraint as adventure.

When it comes to communication and getting a job done, I, in my daily activities, have been subscribing to an overly simplified maxim and usually divide people into two groups: facilitators and complicators. The

---

65 R. Stevens, "Goodbye, Bicentennial: The Recurrent Crisis of Medical Education," New England Journal of Medicine 295, no. 22 (1976) 1252-54.

vocabulary and language invented by the health care administrators is clearly not that of facilitators. Allocation of resources should not be confused with rationing. The common-sense approach to patient care needs to be emphasized and taught in medical schools. A vignette published in the *New England Journal of Medicine* gives me hope and comfort. In it, Drs. Rosenbaum and Lamas wrote the following:

> "Imagine your first medicine rotation. You present a patient admitted overnight with cough, fever, and an infiltrate on chest x-ray. After detailing a history and physical exam you conclude: "This is a 70-year-old man with community-acquired pneumonia. Dead silence. Perhaps, the attending physician says. but *what else* could it be?
>
> Your face reddens. Pulmonary embolism, you say…heart failure.
>
> The patient has a history of asthma. The attending smiles. How might you investigate these other possibilities?And then the two doctors detail the *rule-out* mega-workup, which includes a chest CT scan, echocardiogram, and a multitude of blood tests."[66]

The authors also cite the New York University bioethicist Arthur Caplan: "Can a physician remain a patient advocate while serving as a steward of society's resources?" "The fight about costs is a smokescreen," says Caplan. "What's really at issue is the definition of ethical physician advocacy." I would add: and common sense. A seventy-year-old man with a community-acquired (that is: not complicated by an impairment of the immune system as in patients with AIDS or transplanted organs) pneumonia is treated with IV antibiotics, and the temperature, heart rate, and white blood cell count are monitored. As the patient defervesces and the white cell count drops, he is discharged, and an outpatient clinic follow-up is arranged. In their article, the two physicians continue:

---

66 L. Rosenbaum and D. Laurus, "Cents and Sensitivity—Teaching Physicians to Think about Costs, New England Journal of Medicine, 367, no. 12 (2012) 99-101.

Chris Moriates, a resident at the University of California, San Francisco, has implemented a curriculum for internal medicine residents that teaches them how…to think about cost and how to improve care. Through modules detailing common admission diagnosis, he emphasizes the principles of evidence-based medicine and provides information about associated costs. In one module, a pulmonary embolism develops in a patient. House staff review the tests the patient receives focusing on incremental benefits and associated costs. The patient first undergoes CT angiography at a cost of $3,500. Though the CT shows a pulmonary embolism, house staff subsequently order a D-dimer (a blood test for $450), fibrinogen (another blood test for $100), leg vein Doppler sonography ($1,397) and a full hypercoaguability workup ($2,864). The hospital bill eventually comes to $155,698.…

Now some educational reformers are offering us an added incentive. Put simply, helping a patient become well enough to climb the stairs of his apartment is meaningless if our cure leaves him unable to afford his apartment. Protecting our patients from financial ruin is fundamental to doing no harm Then there is the overtreatment issue. In a recent article in *The New York Times*, the authors said, "American doctors perform a staggering number of tests and procedures, far more than in other industrialized nations. Since 1996, the percentage of doctor visits leading to at least five drugs being prescribed has nearly tripled, and the number of MRI scans had quadrupled. CT scans and MRI scans can lead to false positive results and unnecessary operations, which carry the risk of complications like infections and bleeding. The more medications patients are prescribed, the more likely they are to accidentally overdose or suffer an allergic reaction.

I have noticed over the years that the medication lists of patients have grown longer—some, typewritten, are more than one page long. Some very expensive drugs are clearly not effective, when, for example, the patient continues to smoke a pack of cigarettes a day. Other drugs are being added to treat the side effects of previously prescribed drugs. While many young physicians lack training in the proper management of chronic pain, America is in danger of becoming a "pill nation." Oxycontin is the "hillbilly heroin." There are hundreds of pharmacy robberies each year, and there are "online doctors" who prescribe the oxypills. On the street, they are being sold for $15 to $80 per pill.

In June 2012, the Drug Enforcement Administration (DEA) shut down a ring of pill mills in Miami, Daytona Beach, Jacksonville, Sarasota, Gainesville, and Pensacola. The ring was responsible for thousands of prescriptions and millions of pills. Studies by the Centers for Disease Control (CDC) have found that more people die in the United States every year from prescription drug abuse than from heroin and cocaine (FoxNews.com).

Cardinal Health, a Fortune 500 company, was accused of selling excessive amounts of oxycodone to four Florida pharmacies. Dispensing records show that south Florida pharmacies dispensed thousands of pills to residents of Kentucky and Tennessee who had driven to Florida to visit local doctors (*USA Today*, May 2012). Jeffrey and Christopher George, a team of twin brothers now in prison, had plans to expand their drug-sale operations to Georgia, Missouri, and Texas. They found prescribing doctors on Craigslist; the doctors were paid a flat fee of $75 to $100 per prescription. Apparently, over the two years of their business activities, the brothers made $40 million. In 2010, the amount of prescription drug pain killers sold in Florida and Nevada was in excess of 8.5 kg per 10,000 inhabitants (Bloomberg BusinessWeek).

Why do doctors prescribe these pills, the "oxypills"? Do they fear to be labeled as bad, non-compassionate doctors on web-based rating sites?[67] Pain management is important, as I have pointed out, and difficult. Perhaps the time constraints on the physician and the incentive to see more patients, combined with the never-ending advertisements everyone sees on TV, have led to a quick-fix or "fast food" prescribing culture in which little thought is given to this phenomenon that we share with lab animals called "addiction."

---

67 S. Gupta, "More Treatment, More Mistakes," The New York Times, July 31, 2012.

Chapter 21

Disadvantaged and Worse

Medical students nowadays are being taught about health care disparities and minority diseases—for example, sickle cell disease, which in the United States is a genetic disease of Americans of African descent. For a more complete description of the health care landscape, we need to pay attention to health care disparities and minority diseases.

The problem surfaces on two levels. One issue is that in the African American population, a number of diseases, like high blood pressure and heart disease, take a much more severe and progressive course when compared to the diseases of white patients. The other issue is limited access to and use of health care, which causes delayed recognition and late treatments of diseases. Delayed diagnosis and treatment are not the purview of minorities but problems facing the great numbers of uninsured in this country.

For unclear reasons, African Americans can develop a malignant form of hypertension that is difficult to control and sets these patients up for strokes, heart attacks, and kidney diseases requiring dialysis treatment as early as age forty-five. The benefits of controlling blood pressure are very obvious, but overall we are not yet doing a great job achieving this goal. Often obesity, salty food, and lack of exercise are in the way. Scleroderma, an autoimmune disease, is more severe in blacks than in whites.[68] There are many health care disparities. There is a greater incidence of lung cancer in African American men; breast cancer diagnosis is delayed among African American women; and African American and Hispanic citizens have poorer access to kidney transplantation.[69]African Americans, Hispanics, and

---

68 A. Lembke, "Why Doctors Prescribe Opoids to Known Opoid Abusers," New England Journal of Medicine, 367, no. 17 (2012), 1580-81.
69 R.M. Silver, et al., "Racial Differences between Blacks and Whites with Systemic Sclerosis," Curr Opin Rheumatology (2012).

low-median-income patients are less likely to receive thrombolysis treatment for a stroke,[70] and children with cystic fibrosis who have low-income parents are less likely to receive a lung transplant. One study conducted in the state of Wisconsin found that the disparities in colon cancer incidence and mortality between African American and whites are large and have increased over the last decade. Possibly African Americans are less likely to receive appropriate screening for colon cancer.[71,72]

Awareness of these healthcare disparities—more severe and more progressive disease and delayed diagnosis and treatment as causes of bad outcomes in patients from racial and ethnic minority groups—requires preventive measures and badly needed research into why the disease is worse for some people than others.

---

70 S. Joshi, et al., "Review of Ethnic Disparities in Access to Renal Transplantation," Clinical Transplantation (2012).

71 M.M. Kimball, et al., "Race and Income Disparity in Ischemic Stroke Care: Nationwide Inpatient Sample Database, 2002–2008, J Stroke Cerebrovasc Dis (2012).

72 N.K. LoConte, et al., "Increasing Disparity in Colorectal Cancer Incidence and Mortality among African Americans and Whites: A State's Experience, J. Gastrointest. Oncology (2011).

Chapter 22

Profitable Networking—Is It Profitable to Treat This Condition?

The only valid purpose of a firm is to create a customer.
Peter Drucker

HCA (Hospital Corporation of America) was cofounded in 1968 by two physicians—father Thomas Frist, Sr., and his son, William Frist (the former US Senate majority leader). The system merged in the 1990s with the Columbia Healthcare Corporation, a hospital group led by Rick Scott, who is currently the governor of Florida. A news report from HCA on 2012 second-quarter earnings said that revenues increased 11.9 percent to $8.1 billion, and net income attributable to HCA Holdings, Inc., totaled $391 million. Adjusted EBITDA (earnings before interest, taxes, depreciation, and amortization) increased 10.5 percent to $1.56 billion. HCA has "leading EBITDA MDs," most profitable physicians, and the revenue growth in the second quarter of 2012 was driven by increased patient volume and the consolidation of the HealthONE venture. HCA controls 163 hospitals.

According to an article in *The New York Times* written by Julie Creswell and Reed Abelson in August 2012, HCA has been able to charge more money for the same service and to reduce emergency room overcrowding and expenses by turning away patients with minor conditions like flu or a sprained wrist, unless those patients paid in advance, and by cutting staff costs. HCA is currently under investigation for "generating unnecessary high-cost cardiology services." HCA was purchased in 2006 by Bain Capital, Merrill Lynch, and Kohlberg Kravis Roberts and Company.

Recently in the *New Yorker*, Dr. Atul Gawande compared chain restaurants like The Cheesecake Factory and Red Lobster with chain hospitals. "Hospitals and clinics have been forming into large conglomerates. And physicians—who, facing escalating demands to lower costs, adopt expensive information technology—have been looking to join them. According to the Bureau of Labor Statistics, only a quarter of doctors are now self-employed—an extraordinary turnabout from a decade ago, when a majority were independent."

Dr. Gawande is a surgeon employed by Partners Health Care, which owns Massachusetts General Hospital at Harvard. He describes recent developments in ICU care:

AICU, command center...was outfitted with millions of dollars worth of technology. Banks of computer screens carried live feed of cardiac-monitor readings, radiology-imaging scans, and laboratory results from ICU patients.... Software monitored the stream and produced yellow and red alerts when it detected patterns that raised concerns. Doctors and nurses manned consoles where they could toggle on high-definition video cameras that allowed them to zoom into any ICU room and talk directly to the staff on the scene or to the patients themselves.

He goes on to say, "The concept of the remote ICU started with an effort to let specialists in critical-care medicine, who are in short supply, cover not just one but several community hospitals.... Two hundred and fifty hospitals from Alaska to Virginia have installed a version of the tele-ICU."

Dr. Gawande does not hide that this form of Big Brother medicine is not universally endorsed: "Clinicians have been known to place a gown over the camera.... Remote monitoring will never be the same as being at the bedside." I agree—when in doubt, see the patient. Gawande is impressed with the effective management of the big chain restaurants. They are decidedly "for profit," and he hopes that health care chain operations will likewise become effective when it comes to access and quality of care delivered per dollar. He writes:

"Those of us who work in the health care chains will have to contend with new protocols and technology rollouts every six months, supervisors and project managers and detailed metrics on our performance. Patients won't just look for the best specialist anymore;

they'll look for the best system. Nurses and doctors will have to get used to delivering care in which our own convenience counts for less and the patients' experience for more. We'll also have to figure out how to reward people for taking the time and expense to teach the next generation of clinicians.... The Cheesecake Factory model represents our best prospect for change. Some will see danger in this".[73]

Indeed, employed doctors not following orders can be fired. There is my view of a landscape in a bubble. It will be necessary to look into the bubble from the outside and—in this scenario of industrialized medicine— to put technology-based medicine in its proper place. Historically, modern American medicine has its roots in Europe. Every one of the fathers of American medicine, including Johns Hopkins's William Osler, trained for some time in Europe; Osler visited Berlin and Vienna. Eric Kandel, a Nobel laureate, received the prize for his pioneering work on memory. His book *The Age of Insight* recreates the time and place of modern medicine's origins at the turn of the nineteenth century in Austria. The Vienna physicians insisted on autopsies and began to match the pathology with symptoms and clinical observation. William Osler and others imported these practices to America. After the Second World War, American medicine had established an enormous self-confidence and developed the image of a medicine superpower. Foreign-trained physicians were considered second-class, inferior by training, not properly educated—not up to the standards of American medicine. But during the last decades, medicine, like the economy, has become global. Biomedical research in many European countries, and in Japan and China, is booming and frequently better funded than medical research in the United States. European doctors ask, "How is it possible that the superpower America has so many uninsured patients? Why does America not have a better health care system? It will be worthwhile to look at the AHCI from the outside of the bubble.

The traditional hierarchical organization of the medical schools, which provide the training of the physicians, with departments, divisions, sections, and a pecking order of residents, interns and students, provides marching

---

73 Gawande A. "Big Med", The New Yorker, August 13, 2012.

orders and generates physicians who obey orders—not trouble makers. A critical analysis of the system by American doctors—from within this system—is difficult and almost always self-referential. New technology and new regulations imposed on the physicians are rarely questioned as Dr. Gawande so poignantly describes. Fatalism in the ranks of the physicians is widespread, and there are now signs that things are not well. There is professional burnout. Apparently, doctors in America can't work in The Cheesecake Factory anymore. Research over the last ten years has shown that burnout—"the particular constellation of emotional exhaustion, detachment, and a low sense of accomplishment—is widespread among medical students and doctors in training." Dr. Tait Shanafelt is the lead author of a Mayo Clinic-initiated study based on the analysis of questionnaires sent to more than seven thousand doctors. The researchers compared the responses of the doctors with those of 3,500 people working in other professions and found, after adjusting for gender, age, and number of hours worked, that the doctors were more likely to suffer from burnout. More than half of the doctors in family medicine, emergency medicine and general internal medicine experience some form of burnout. A significant number of doctors feel trapped, stymied by the ever-changing rules and regulations. Some feel guilty because they are not allowed the time to work up all the problems on the "problem list"—one problem per visit, they are being told. They don't like to be told by insurers and other payers what they can prescribe, and they are frustrated when they hear their patients saying: "I can't afford this medication." Dr. Shanafelt says, "Doctors are losing their inspiration. Doctors who are frustrated and burned out are likely to quit, to stop practicing. " If people work in an environment in which they are seeing no meaning, no purpose—people who joined the profession and answered the call to help patients, not to make money for The Cheesecake Factory—they will step out.

In the old days, I used to attend in the medical ICU for one month straight with no weekend off. At the end of the month, a long weekend of camping and hiking in the Rocky Mountain National Park would do wonders. I think I never experienced burnout. Things are different now: There are revolving-door admissions and discharges and administrators who tell you (sometimes triumphantly) what you *can't* do. That part I have been taking badly. The system has degenerated to a "can't do" system. Worst of all, the outlook, the future, is bleak. But we can't let computer banks and plain-clothes regulators destroy the medical profession.

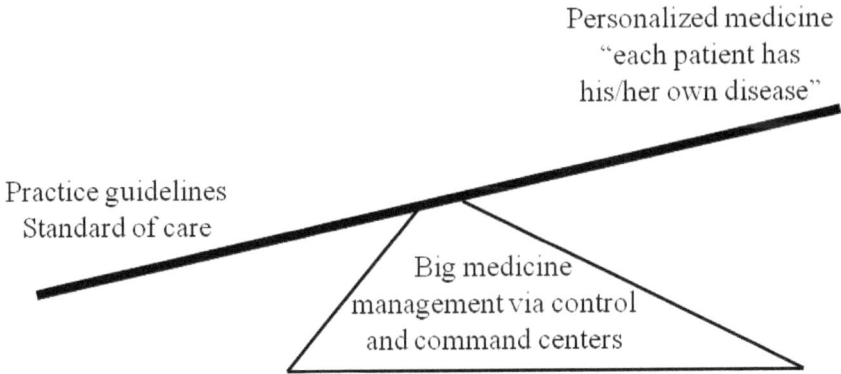

Personalized medicine
"each patient has
his/her own disease"

Practice guidelines
Standard of care

Big medicine
management via control
and command centers

Chapter 23

A Conversation with Dr. Sharon Rounds

A survey of the American health care system would be incomplete without a brief discussion of the Veterans Administration (VA) facilities. President Hoover created the Veterans Administration in 1930. By 1947 there were ninety seven hospitals in operation. Now there are 152 hospitals, 800 community based outpatient clinics and 126 nursing homes (source: Department of Veterans Affairs, April 2012). In order to get information about the health care provided by the VA system , I called Dr. Sharon Rounds.

NFV: Greetings, Sharon, and thanks for making time for this conversation, I know how busy you are running the medical service at the VA hospital, running your lab, writing grants—and then, in addition, being pestered by me to write a perspective on the effects of cigarette smoking on lung cells. But I hope that you can quickly answer some questions in regards to the workings of the VA Health Care System. As you know, Americans have little understanding of what socialism is, how it works, and in these politically charged times, the specter of socialism, socialized medicine, etc., is constantly being raised. From a European perspective, the VA health care system can be seen as a highly successful experiment in social medicine. Let me stop here and find out whether you agree.

SR (Sharon Rounds, Chief of Medical Service, Providence VA Medical Center, Providence, RI): Well, I must say, I struggle a bit with this concept. I guess perhaps I never thought about the VA in these terms. When we were fellows in training, we just took care of patients and brought our chest x-ray films and cases to Marvin Schwarz's Friday x-ray conference to be

With regard to your question about "social medicine," I am not sure that I know what "socialized medicine" is! I would characterize the VA as a large, single-payer, managed-care health system that cares for a special group of individuals who earned their health care by service to their country.

The VA does a terrific job with health care, as assessed by the same objective criteria as Medicare. The VA underwent a huge transformation in the 1990s that remarkably improved the quality of health care. You should take a look at the book by Phillip Longman, *Best Care Anywhere: Why VA Healthcare Is Better Than Yours.*[73] Longman makes the point that because veterans sign up for lifelong health care, the VA can take the long-range view, and it becomes cost-effective to actually prevent disease. Also, VA physicians are salaried by the VA, so there is no incentive for doctors to perform unnecessary procedures. Indeed, efficient care is rewarded by the salary bonus system. Finally, the VA embraced information technology years before other parts of the US healthcare system with an electronic medical record designed by clinicians, rather than by accountants. The EMR allows the VA to monitor and measure outcomes of care and to provide physicians feedback and incentives to improve healthcare.

NFV: Sharon, I looked at the Providence VA website to learn about access to care in the VA system, and I am interested to find out who pays for what. I read that the Veterans Health Administration provides care for about 8.3 million veterans per year, that the VA has an online prescription service, and that it provides dental care—the latter as one-time dental care within 180 days of discharge from the service. What I am particularly interested in is what kind of care veterans can receive when their disease is not service-connected. There is a wonderful video that takes you step by step through the application process for VA health care. A friendly female voice explains that veterans need to reveal their total household income and that copayments may have to be made—and also that enrollment in the VA health care can be denied. Unfortunately, I was unable to find the enrollment criteria online. Can you help me with this?

SR: If a veteran has health insurance, then the VA will charge the insurance but not bill the veteran for uncovered expenses. Copayments apply to several services and are very reasonable, based on income and whether their disability is related to their active duty time in the armed services. Some

---

73 Phillip Longman, Best Care Anywhere: Why VA Healthcare Is Better Than Yours (Sausalito, CA: PoliPoint Press, 2007).

patients have no copay at all. Care provided as part of a VA research project does not require a copayment.

NFV: It looks to me that the VA health care is very comprehensive; it also includes hospice care and in-home aides. Whether we call that socialism or not, I guess you agree that the system works for the patients and their families—not many veterans fall through the cracks.... Once in a while, I encounter a homeless person on a street corner flashing a cardboard sign reading: "Disabled veteran. Everything helps! God Bless." My question is: Are there homeless veterans without access to the VA? I had understood that they receive support when they are disabled.

SR: You are correct—because the VA provides comprehensive care, as a clinician I can arrange for appropriate services for my patients very easily. However, for the purposes of VA health benefits and services, someone dishonorably discharged is not considered eligible for VA health care. That is where the line is drawn, but once a veteran is enrolled, that veteran remains enrolled. The VA health care system has not been designed with profit making in mind, so deductibles are very reasonable, calculated according to the veteran's income.

Traditionally, the VA primarily serviced males. However, with more and more women serving in the military, the Women Veterans Program has been vastly expanded from primary care to treatments of all chronic illnesses.

The VA has also developed a terrific system for working with homeless veterans that started with pilot projects and now is being promulgated throughout the VA system. Let me give you an example of how the Homeless Veterans Program works to improve health and reduce expensive hospitalizations. I recently saw a patient with Chronic Obstructive Pulmonary Disease (COPD) who had been hospitalized four times in as many months at our VA for exacerbations of his lung disease. I realized that he was homeless and that he had some alcohol-use issues. I called the Homeless Veteran Office; they made contact with the gentleman (not so easy with the homeless!), helped him sober up, found him housing, and helped him keep clinic appointments. He has not been hospitalized now for the past two years!

NFV: Having been brought up during my formative years in Europe, I have noticed early on that the term "socialized" in the United States is usually uttered as a pejorative, and most commonly in the context of publically funded health care.

SR: People who work for the veterans' health care system do not regard it as "socialized medicine" but rather as an opportunity to work in an environment in which the physician is not driven to provide "more" but rather to provide appropriate and efficient health care. Frankly, I would not be surprised if the VA did not become a model for single-payer systems in the future.

NFV: Thanks for your time and help, Sharon.

Chapter 24

Medical Care in the Netherlands—A Model for US Reform?

Let us briefly move out of the bubble and examine a different healthcare system, the Dutch system.

The Dutch reformed their health care system rather recently, in 2006. The Netherlands's population is 16.7 million (a bit more than double the population of Virginia); the country, because of its former colonies, in particular Indonesia, is multi-ethnic. The Dutch health care system is organized in three compartments. The first compartment deals with the coverage of long-term chronic illness care, paid by income-related contributions (12.55 percent of taxable income) and a general government revenue grant. The second compartment deals with essential medical care delivered by general practitioners and short-term hospital stays. The third compartment deals with supplementary care like dental work, physiotherapy, and cosmetic surgery. Patients buy supplementary insurance for the procedures not covered by the basic Social Health Insurance.

The "basic package" offered by insurers details the reasonable costs and is defined by the Dutch government to include the following:

- General practitioner appointments, hospital care, and prescribed specialist care
- Dentistry for children and young adults, specialist dentistry and dentures for those older than 18
- Ambulance services
- Postnatal care
- Certain medications
- Rehabilitative services
- Quit-smoking programs

All individuals are required to purchase the basic health care package or face a fine worth 130 percent of the premium. Insurers are obligated to accept any application; they cannot complicate access or deny coverage. Individuals can choose between fourteen Dutch health care insurers and can receive tax credits that make the package affordable to patients with low income.

Dutch citizens contribute to the Social Health Insurance system a flat-rate premium—directly to the insurer of their choice—of €1,065 per year (2009 coverage). This constitutes about 50 percent of the Dutch health care funding. The government covers the cost of health care for children and some of the health care costs of illegal immigrants. Every Dutch citizen is required to register with a family practitioner who acts as a navigator and gatekeeper to control costs by limiting referrals to specialists.

More than 90 percent of Dutch hospitals are managed on a not-for-profit basis, and, as of 2007, insurance companies can negotiate prices on 20 percent of the services.

A few numbers are necessary to provide perspective:

- Unemployment rate in the Netherlands : 4.4 percent (2011 estimate)
- Labor force: 7.8 million
- Population below the poverty line: 10.5 percent (2005 estimate),
- Out-of-pocket expenses for medical bills of more than $1,000 per year: 5 percent (United States: 30 percent)

Clearly, Holland is a small country, however the Dutch economy is the fifth largest in the Euro-zone and the Dutch apparently can afford a uniform health care coverage system.

Is it really that simple? Or are there factors and conditions that make the Netherlands not a model for American uniform health care reform?

The Dutch system provides universal access and consumer choice of insurance. Patients in America struggle with both issues. While it is unclear whether the Dutch system can work only in a small country and cannot be upscaled to the size of the U.S. population, the Dutch health-care system is not a Medicare volunteer system that, when proposed in the United States, was called "Social Darwinism" (President Obama) or "right-wing social engineering" (Newt Gingrich). While the US health care problem is aesthetically displeasing and morally reprehensible, other countries that rather recently established a national health care coverage system, like Taiwan (population:21.1 million people), in 1995, chose a National Health Insurance system, which, since 2004, covers 99 percent of all citizens. The per capita health expenditure in 2000 totaled $752. Interestingly, the Taiwanese modeled their National Health Insurance after Medicare in the United States—only the Taiwanese system covers everyone, not just the elderly.

Chapter 25

Big and Not-So-Big Pharma

Prostacyclin is a lipid molecule that is made by the endothelium—the innermost layer of cells covering the lumen of blood vessels. It was discovered by Sir John Vane, who was awarded the Nobel Prize for this discovery in 1971. Prostacyclin is one of the most powerful vasodilators known to man and very effectively relaxes the lung blood vessels. Burroughs Wellcome, the former British pharmaceutical giant (now part of Glaxo) had synthesized this molecule, which has a very rapid onset of action and is also quickly metabolized and inactivated. Because of these properties, prostacyclin was soon used in the heart catheter lab to test whether, in patients, the pulmonary hypertension was fixed (unresponsive to vasodilator drugs) or whether the pulmonary artery pressure during an infusion of prostacyclin could drop. This test is important because patients who have a significant drop of their pressure have a better outcome and can be treated relatively easily. Although prostacyclin must be infused continuously by a pump, it was initially tested in patients with heart failure, and the treatment trial was unsuccessful (the heart failure trial was stopped prematurely). For a while, prostacyclin was a drug in search of a disease. At that time, lung transplantation or heart/lung transplantation was the only effective treatment for severe pulmonary arterial hypertension. Tim Higenbottam, then a member of the lung transplant team at Papworth Hospital in Cambridge, England, and a creative investigator, had the idea in 1984 to treat a young woman, bedbound with severe pulmonary hypertension with continuous intravenous infusion of prostacyclin, which enabled her to live independently at home for thirteen months—until she received a transplant. As we say, the rest is history, and in the spirit of my mentor, Jack Reeves, who used to say: "Randomize the first case—*to treatment*," Tim had just done that.

I began to see patients with severe pulmonary hypertension in 1981 at the University of Colorado Medical Center in Denver at a time when the median survival of so-called primary or idiopathic pulmonary hypertension after the diagnosis was 2.8 years, (which, statistically speaking, meant that three years after the diagnosis, 50 percent of the patients had died). It's a disease worse than many cancers. In these years, two of my patients made it to heart/lung transplantation. Robin Barst, a pediatric cardiologist at Columbia University in New York, convinced Sir John that prostacyclin needed to be tried as a long-term treatment for primary pulmonary hypertension, and in 1994 she published a paper stating that prostacyclin treatment resulted in lasting improvement and that a few of the initially treated eighteen patients survived longer than sixty months. The conclusion of the investigator team was that "long-term prostacyclin may be especially helpful in seriously ill patients awaiting transplantation." Two years earlier, in 1992, based on Tim Higenbottam's single case report, David Badesch and I asked the University Hospital Institutional Review Board (IRB) to give us a "compassionate use" approval to treat a twenty-nine-year-old woman with idiopathic pulmonary hypertension and end-stage right heart failure with continuous prostacyclin. The IRB gave us approval, and within twenty-four hours, Burroughs-Wellcome shipped the drug, and we started treating the young woman. A miracle happened. A day after we started the drug, the patient improved; one week later, she walked out of the hospital. That was our unforgettable first successfully treated patient. The systematic treatment with prostacyclin treatment had to wait until FDA approval of the drug for idiopathic pulmonary hypertension, which followed Robin Barst's *New England Journal of Medicine* paper in 1996.

Prostacyclin (also known as epoprostenol) was and is prohibitively expensive; it costs about $100,000 per year. Although prostacyclin treatment does not cure the disease, many patients have survived with the continuous infusion therapy for more than fifteen years. Our young patient's treatment success made it clear that we had experienced the first breakthrough in the treatment of severe pulmonary hypertension and that this expensive and difficult treatment (the patient has to learn how to mix the drug in a sterile environment, fill a cassette, and program a pump) required special attention. We advertised this new treatment option by mailing letters to all the pulmonologists and cardiologists in the state of Colorado. I approached the dean of the medical school with the proposal to form a multidisciplinary Pulmonary Hypertension Center. By 1993, we brought physicians and investigators from the divisions of pulmonary medicine, cardiology, rheumatology, and immunology and from the departments of pathology and pharmacology together to study pulmonary hypertension as a team. The center became a success. Patients were referred and traveled from Montana, Wyoming, and New Mexico–the Rocky Mountain corridor–to the Pulmonary Hypertension Center in Denver for diagnosis and treatment. The pathologists used new technologies to identify the abnormal cells in the lung vessels. Animal lungs were analyzed, and new drugs were tried in experimental models. The American daughter company of Schering in Berlin, Berlex, had developed a much longer biologically active prostacyclin analogue called iloprost, so we started to lobby the company to develop this drug for pulmonary hypertension. They did not want to do this.

We sent letters to Berlin with pleas to develop the drug. Schering said that the American daughter had grown up and made her decisions independently. I thought that the proof of successful treatment with prostacyclin would encourage the pharma industry to develop other drugs for pulmonary hypertension. I started to visit several companies and made my case for pulmonary hypertension drug development. Usually, after I had finished my talk, in the question-and-answer session, people from the marketing division would say, "Let's assume that we have a pulmonary hypertension drug. Do you think that in the first year of sales our revenue would be more or less than fifty million?" I did not have an answer to this question. The size of the national or international market was completely unknown.

In 1995, I was invited by a husband and wife team of investigators to visit one of the large Swiss pharma concerns. They had been working with a compound that blocked the recently discovered endothelin receptors. (Endothelin is a small protein produced by endothelial cells and a powerful vasoconstrictor substance.) When asked what I thought about the potential of an endothelial receptor blocker for pulmonary hypertension treatment, I said that it was difficult for me to envision that there would be one single mediator or factor that caused human pulmonary hypertension and that the proof would be in the clinical pudding. In 1996, the pharma team in Switzerland published their first paper. It showed, in a model of chronic pulmonary hypertension, that the endothelin receptor blocker had reduced the pulmonary artery pressure by 13 percent, and they suggested that endothelin plays a causal role in pulmonary hypertension.

As the big pharma company decided not to develop the drug for treatment of high blood pressure or chronic congestive heart failure, the entrepreneurial husband and wife team formed their own company and began to sponsor clinical trials testing the effect of their drug in patients with severe pulmonary hypertension. The first-placebo-controlled trial of the receptor blocker was published in 2002. Since then, the FDA approved pill has been prescribed for thousands of patients worldwide. This drug was the first orally active pulmonary hypertension drug. It changed the way we treat pulmonary hypertension, and many clinical trials followed. That was the heyday of the pulmonary hypertension trialists (groups of doctors who design and conduct the clinical studies). Soon, another drug was discovered to show an effect in pulmonary hypertension trials. Practically all of the diagnosed patients now are registered and enrolled in one or another of the many ongoing clinical trials.

The industry was initially astonished. There was indeed a market for pulmonary hypertension drugs, and as the years have gone on, some pulmonary hypertension centers have several study coordinators employed and are administering five, seven, and ten study protocols simultaneously. If patients were excluded from participating in one study, they were likely eligible for another study.

Study costs are calculated per enrolled patient, and this (for hospitals) revenue-generating research—the studies cost millions—produces the data required for drug approval and for marketing. The trialists write papers about the drug or the drug combinations. But there is a downside to this. The trialists are so busy running the studies for the industry that they have no time to think about the disease itself. The drugs do not cure the disease. There are treatment responders and non-responders. Who responds to a particular treatment, and why, remains unclear and has not been studied. As patients continue to die from pulmonary hypertension, the treating physicians have not formed an international multicenter team of investigators who join hands to figure out the root causes of severe pulmonary hypertension. A member of the NIH Lung Division summed it up nicely: "The problem with your patients is that they are very expensive—and then they die anyway."

Dr.Alejandro Macchia and his group of coworkers analyzed a large number of clinical pulmonary hypertension trials. They concluded that the treatment benefits were confined only to patients with advanced disease and only for a sixteen-week treatment period—the duration of the studies—and that the impact of vasodilators on long-term patient survival remains uncertain. In an update one year later, Macchia and coauthors wrote the following: "Further studies utilizing similar classes of drugs...are unlikely to yield different results or offer any more clinical benefits. Given that pulmonary arterial hypertension is a fatal disease, this raises concerns about whether they (these trials) are ethical to conduct or not."

Where do we go from here?

We need new drugs and a method to identify the patients responding to treatment—and why. We can't just go on doing what we have been doing for the last ten years. I like to remind the reader that all of the drugs we use today for the treatment of pulmonary hypertension were not designed for the treatment of pulmonary hypertension. Prostacyclin, after it had been synthesized, was supposed to treat congestive heart failure, so was the first endothelin receptor blocker. The drug most recently added to the repertoire was developed for the treatment of erectile dysfunction! In one way or the other, all three groups of drugs entered the pulmonary hypertension market through the back door of "off-label use."

The way forward is to learn the lessons from cancer research: Understand the biology of the cells involved in the disease—and then develop a target. Some believe that idiopathic pulmonary hypertension is not a disease that begins and ends in the lung. When established, it is likely a disease in which there is involvement of the bone marrow, the immune system, and the endocrine system. That means a systems biology approach will be required. Using vasodilator drugs is akin to the man who lost his house key in the night, searching for the key in the small illuminated circle under the lamppost—because that's where the light is.

Will the pharmaceutical industry now make an honest effort to understand the nuts and bolts of pulmonary hypertension and invest in new drug development? Or will they continue to sell the expensive, old drugs (to increase their market share) that we now know have a limited impact on the disease? The business end of all of this remains opaque and problematic. If Dr. Macchia is only partially correct with his assessment, the latter is the likely scenario.

Chapter 26

A Virtual Conversation about the Prospects of Health Care Reform in America

This conversation did not really take place but could have if Tom Petty, one of the pioneering American lung doctors, were still alive today.

NFV: Tom, you had your share of health care experience: three mitral valve replacements, endocarditis (inflammation of heart valves), and kidney failure. I know you have your own thoughts about the American health care system. Over the years, you collected articles that address health care issues, patient care, and patient–doctor relationships. I wonder what your position would be today and how you envision that America gets out of this health care dilemma. What has happened lately in America? What kind of medicine are we practicing now in the twenty-first century? You left a folder behind with articles addressing health care reform, and comments, but unfortunately no notes. You had put a label on the folder that asks "What is wrong with medicine?" I am trying to figure out what your opinion is about American medicine and health care today.

TLP (Thomas L. Petty, the former head of the Pulmonary and Critical Care Division at the Health Sciences Center of the University of Colorado): I can't say that my experience with my illness, the surgeries, the defibrillator, and the other nuisances that made the last years of my life miserable was a good one. If you believe that I was in charge of my health care, you are wrong. I tried to be, but most of the time things happened to me and I had to deal with them. What irked me most was the lack of a common-sense approach.

I have noticed that there are now a lot of health care experts who know the numbers of everything and write a lot. They write about the state of healthcare and the "status syndrome" with the opening line "The poor have poor health" But, frankly, I am unsure what these experts really know. They write about the strengthening of primary care. ·It's like whistling in the

141

dark forest. They predict a physician shortage in six or seven years in the United States and describe the geography of medically underserved communities—in other words, the boonies.... I wonder whether the experts see the big picture. As you know, we can see a lot through the bronchoscope, but we can also see some things with the retrospectoscope.

NFV: Tom, you always said about our work as physicians: "If we can't do it well, we are not doing it at all!" How are you applying this principle today, where many doctors know that they can't do the best job they want to do—and feel guilty about it?

TLP: Yes, I used to say that. And I meant it, too. Having been a sick physician has been the worst experience. Of course, "Physician, heal yourself!" does not work. Before I had my heart surgeries, I felt that our health care system was OK, but being at the other end of the stethoscope taught me otherwise. I clearly handled the doctor part much better than the patient part. There were too many moments when I needed to call the shots and could not.

NFV: You once drafted a plan/agenda for ambulatory care training in internal medicine. Under the headline "How to become a real doctor," you wrote the following:

- Dealing with the symptoms
- Clinical problem solving
- Health promotion
- Cost savings/effectiveness in office practice
- Methods of referral/communication/courtesy/feedback
- Dealing with third-party payers/insurances
- Planning for the future/living will/durable power
- Assisting the patient in self-management

TLP: Yes, and then I quoted from the AMA's (American Medical Association's) 2001 statement: A physician shall, while caring for a patient, regard responsibly to the patient as paramount, and, a physician shall support access to medical care for all people.

NFV: That was ten years ago.
TLP: True!

142

Chapter 27

Recommendations for Baby Boomers

The following are some suggestions to help Baby Boomers stay healthy.
- Try to stay active.
- Exercise your body and your brain. As you age, your muscles get weaker. You need your quadriceps and your triceps to get out of the chair! If you do not exercise, soon you will not be able to put your socks on or tie your shoelaces. Exercise increases the blood flow through the brain and has been shown to preserve memory function. Weight lifting is now recommended for stroke rehabilitation. Read, learn something new, and learn a new language before your horizon and the field of your activities starts to narrow and all your friends die.
- Make new friends! Take your life partner out to a surprise dinner!
- Walk!
- Spend time with your grandchildren!
- Get your house in order—and please do not leave the process of medical decision making to guesswork or tacit assumptions. Have an advance directive or living will, and let your family know where to find this document.
- Be interested in your insurance status. Find out what your copayments are.
- Find a doctor who will inform you and tell you the whole truth.
- Medications are necessary for the control of high blood pressure, diabetes, and asthma, but often, fewer pills are better. Know your copayments!
- Gastric reflux, sleep apnea, and diabetes (type II) improve with weight loss, which can result from a smart diet and exercise.
- Life is hills and valleys; try to stay somewhere between!

Easily said.

Acknowledgments

I would like to thank the early readers of the manuscript: Maria and Don Johnson, Sandra Dingus, and Barbara Jacobi. I also wish to thank my former research associate and friend Mark Nicolls, a fellow pulmonologist from Stanford University who read the manuscript and "got it." I want to thank Sharon Rounds, the Chief of Medicine at the Veterans Hospital in Providence, Rhode Island, for discussions and helpful advice. Louise Nett, who watched my first baby steps in pulmonary medicine, sent me Tom Petty's folder with his health care articles. Harm Bogaard, Vrije Universiteit of Amsterdam, fact-checked my description of the Dutch Health Care System. My assistant, Peyton Stroud, did the hard work and never grew impatient with my endless changes and additions. Jose Gomez Arroyo helped with the cover design. My wife, Angelika, supported me throughout our life together, even when I was collecting frequent-flier miles and, for many years, was largely an absentee father who wrote grant applications and papers rather than watching our daughter's field hockey games on Saturdays. A literary agent wrote me that doctors' memoirs are difficult to sell these days and "to be salable, they need to have a context beyond the immediate experiences of the narrator, a context of the greater world that looms around us." Very good. I won't worry about the greater context, as long as the view on the greater landscape remains unobstructed and the readers appreciate the politics of the bubble. My hope is to have provided just enough of the facts about the AHCI and that I have been somewhat successful staying away from polemics and preaching. I never intended to write a memoir as characterized by the literary agents. Rereading John Steinbeck's *Travels with Charley*, published in 1962, and based on a road trip through pre- civil-rights-movement America, gave me the format for *When in Doubt, See the Patient*, a string of short essays. Each essay is a signpost in the American healthcare landscape, which the reader can use for orientation. The short essay encourages what one of my former mentors has called "economy of words."

Working for the plaintiff, the patient, and "economy of words" has guided me through the years of my travels.

Sources

Chapter 1
I Think I Can't Afford My Disease

Iglehart, J.K. "Expanding Eligibility, Cutting Costs—A Medicaid Update. *New England Journal of Medicine* 366, no. 12 (2012): 105–107.

Mirnezami R, J. Nicholson, and A. Darzi. "Preparing for Precision Medicine." *New England Journal of Medicine* 366, no. 6 (2012): 489–9 1.

Murray J.F. "Personalized Medicine: Been There, Done That, Always Needs Work." *American Journal of Respiratory Critical Care Medicine* 185, no. 2 (2012) 1251–52.

Further Reading

Pollack, A. "Sanofi Halves Price of Cancer Drug Zaltrap after Sloan-Kettering Rejection." *The New York Times*, November 8, 2012.

Chapter 2
A Short Overview of the History of Health Insurance in America

Blendon, R.J., et al. "Understanding Health Care in the 2012 Election." *New England Journal of Medicine* 367, no. 17 (October 2012): 1658–61.

David, M.M. "The American Approach to Health Insurance." *The Milbank Memorial Fund Quarterly* (1934).

Davis, K. "Universal Coverage in the United States: Lessons from Experience of the Twentieth Century." *Journal of Urban Health: Bulletin of the New York Academy of Medicine* (2001).

Fitch, S.S. *Six Lectures on the Function of the Lungs.* New York: J.H. Mackenzie, 1862.

Light, D.W. "Historical and Comparative Reflections on the US National Health Insurance Reforms." *Social Science and Medicine* (2011).

McGill, M. "Human Rights from the Grassroots Up: Vermont's Campaign for Universal Health Care." *Health Human Rights* (2012).

Starr, P. *The Social Transformation of American Medicine.* New York: Basic, 1982.

Further Reading

Fineberg, H.V., "Shattuck Lecture: A Successful and Sustainable Health System—How to Get There from Here." *New England Journal of Medicine* 366, no. 11 (2012): 1020–27.

Lee, T.H. "Care Redesign—A Path Forward for Providers." *New England Journal of Medicine* 367, no. 5 (2012): 466–72.

Obama, Barack. "Securing the Future of American Health Care." *New England Journal of Medicine* 365, no. 15 (2012): 1377–81.

Romney, Mitt. "Replacing Obamacare with Real Health Care Reform. *New England Journal of Medicine* 367, no. 15 (2012): 1377–81.

Chapter 3
Global Payments and Opportunity in Austerity

Baicker, K., and A. Chandra. "The Health Care Jobs Fallacy." *New England Journal of Medicine* 366, no. 26 (2012): 2433–35.

Pizzo, P.A., and N.M. Clark. "Alleviating Suffering 101: Pain Relief in the United States." *New England Journal of Medicine* 366, no. 3 (2012): 197–99.

Skine, N.W., and D.A. Chokshi. "Opportunity in Austerity—A Common Agenda for Medicine and Public Health." *New England Journal of Medicine* 366, no. 5 (2012): 395–97.

Further Reading

Asch, D., and K. Volpp. "What Business Are We In? The Emergence of Health as the Business of Health Care." *New England Journal of Medicine* 367, no. 10 (2012): 888–89.

Fuchs, V.R. "Major Trends in the US Health Economy Since 1950." *New England Journal of Medicine* 366, no. 11 (2012): 973–77.

Marvasti, F.F. and R.S. Stafford, "From Sick Care to Health Care–Reengineering Prevention into the US System." *New England Journal of Medicine* 367, no. 10 (2012): 889–91.

Chapter 4
Bundled Care

Cutler, D.M., and K. Gosh. "Potential for Cost Saving through Bundled Episode Payments." *New England Journal of Medicine* 366, no. 12 (2012): 1075–77.

Jacoby, S. "Taking Responsibility for Death." *The New York Times*, March 30, 2012.

Liptak, A. Justice Anthony M. Kennedy may be Key to Health Ruling *The New York Times*, March 30, 2012.

Van Lare, J.M., and P.H. Conway. "Value-Based Purchasing—National Programs Move from Volume to Value." *New England Journal of Medicine* (2012).

Further Reading

Asch, D.A., R.W. Muller, and K.G. Volpp. "Automated Hovering in Health Care—Watching Over the 5000 Hours." *New England Journal of Medicine* 367, no. 1 (2012): 1–3.

Richman, B.D., M.A. Hall, and K.A. Schulman. "Overbilling and Informed Financial Consent—A Contractual Solution." *New England Journal of Medicine* 367, no. 5 (2012): 396–97.

Chapter 5
The Girl Who Died Twice

Lerner, B.L. "A Case that Shook Medicine." *The Washington Post*, November 2006.

Lerner, B.L. "A Life-Changing Case for Doctors in Training." *The New York Times*, August 2011.

Robins, Natalie S.. "The Girl Who Died Twice." Dell,1996

Further Reading

Kaplan, R.M., J.M. Satterfield, and R.S. Kington. "Building a Better Physician–The Case for the New MCAT." *New England Journal of Medicine* 366, no. 14 (2012): 1265–68.

Truog, R.D. "Patients and Doctors—Evolution of a Relationship." *New England Journal of Medicine* 366, no. 7 (2012): 581–85.

Chapter 6
Only the Hypothesis Enables You to See What Can Be Seen

Adler, L. *Primary Malignant Growth of the Lungs and Bronchi.* London: Longmans,Green and Company, 1912.

Gillum, L.A., et al. "NIH Disease Funding Levels and Burden of Disease." PLoS ONE 2011, be16837.

Goulart, B.H., et al. "Lung cancer screening with low-dose computed tomography. *J Natl Compr Canc. Netw* (2012).

Moore, L,G., and R.F. Grover. "Jack Reeves and His Science." *Physiol Neurobiology* 151, no. 2–3 (2006): 96–108.

Nagrath, et al. "Isolation of Rare Circulating Tumour Cells in Cancer Patients by Microchips Technology." *Nature* 450 (2007): 1235.

Pirie, K., R. Peto, G.K. Reeves, et al. "The Twenty-First Century Hazards of Smoking and Benefits of Stopping: a Prospective Study of One Million Women in the UK." *Lancet* (October 26, 2012).

Further Reading

Peters–Golden, M., J.R. Klinger, and S.S. Carson. "The Case for Increased Funding for Research in Pulmonary and Critical Care." *Am J Respir Crit Care Med* 186, no. 3 (2012): 213–15.

Rohrhoff, N.J. "Becoming a Physician. What Life Is Like." *New England Journal of Medicine* 366, no. 8 (2012): 683–85.

Verghese, A. "Culture Shock—Patient as Icon, Icon as Patient." *New England Journal of Medicine* 359, no. 26 (2008): 2748–51.

Chapter 7
Flat Screens

Chapter 8
Clinician–Scientists and Translational Research

Khadaroo, R.G., and O.D. Rotstein. Are Clinician–Scientists an Endangered Species? Barriers to Clinician–Scientist Training." *Clin Invest Med* 25, no. 6 (2002): 260–61.

Roberts, S.F., et al., "Perspective: Transforming Science into Medicine: How Clinician–Scientists Can Build Bridges Across Research's 'Valley of Death.'" *Accad Med* 87, no. 3 (2012): 266–70.

Further Reading

Gelijns, A.C., and S.E. Gabriel. "Looking Beyond Translation–Integrating Clinical Research with Medical Practice." *New England Journal of Medicine* 366, no. 18 (2012): 1659–61.

Hendrickson, S., and D. Altshuler, "Risk and Return for the Clinician–Investigator." *Sci Transl Med* 4, no. 135 (2012): 135cm6.

Chapter 9
High Colonics, Magnetic Water, and the "Art of Medicine"

Akl, E.A., and H.J. Schunemann. "Routine Heparin for Patients with Cancer? One answer, More Questions." *New England Journal of Medicine* 366, no.7 (2012) 661-2.

Ernst, E. "Colonic Irrigation and the Theory of Autointoxication: A Triumph of Ignorance over Science." *Journal of Clinical Gastroenterology* 4(1997)196-8.

Fanikos, J., et al. "Venous Thromboembolism Prophylaxis for Medical Service—Mostly Cancer—Patients at Hospital Discharge." *Am J Med* 124, no. 12 (2011): 1143–50.

Further Reading

Broad, W.J. "Applying Science to Alternative Medicine." *The New York Times*, September 29, 2008.

Weeks, J.C., et al. "Patients' Expectations about Effects of Chemotherapy for Advanced Cancer." *New England Journal of Medicine* 367, no. 17 (2012): 1616–25.

Chapter 10
The Respirator: A Device to Prolong Life—Not Death

Hobin, J.A., and R.A. Galbraith. "Engaging Basic Scientists in Translational Research." FASEB 26, no. 6 (2012): 2227–30.

Further Reading

Smith, T.J., and D.L. Longo. "Talking with Patients About Dying." *New England Journal of Medicine* 367, no. 17 (2012): 1651–52.

Chapter 11
More Important than Pain: The Desire to Be in Control

Further Reading

Jacoby, S. "Taking Responsibility for Death." *The New York Times*, March 30, 2012.

Lamas, D., and L. Rosenbaum. "Freedom from the Tyranny of Choice– Teaching the End-of-Life Conversation." *New England Journal of Medicine* 366, no. 18 (2012): 1655–57.

Prokopetz, J.J., and L.S. Lehmann. "Redefining Physicians' Role in Assisted Dying." *New England Journal of Medicine* 367, no. 2 (2012) 97-9.

Chapter 12
Comfort Care

Further Reading

Colla, C.H., et al. "Impact of Payment Reform on Chemotherapy at the End of Life. *Am J Manag Care* 18, no. 5 (2012): e200–8.

Stevenson, D.G. "Growing Pains for the Medicare Hospice Benefit." *New England Journal of Medicine* 367, no. 18 (2012): 1683–85.

Chapter 13
Halloween Does Not Do It

Chapter 14
Quality Assessment and Online Reputation Management

Asch, D.A., and K.G. Volpp. "What Businesses Are We In? The Emergence of Health as the Business of Health Care." *New England Journal of Medicine* 367, no. 10 (2012): 888–89.

Calman, N.S., et al. "Lost to Follow-Up: The Public Health Goals of Accountable Care." *Arch Intern Med* 172, no. 7 (2012): 584–86.

Gourevitch, M.N., et al. "The Challenge of Attributions: Responsibility for Population Health in the Context of Accountable Care." *Am J Public Health* 42, no. 6, 2 (2012): 5180–83.

Jones, D., et al. "The Burden of Disease and the Changing Task of Medicine. *New England Journal of Medicine* 366, no. 25 (2012): 2333–38.

Kellermann, A.L., et al. "Emergency Departments, Medicaid Costs, and Access to Primary Care—Understanding the Link." *New England Journal of Medicine* 366, no. 23 (2012): 2141–43.

Further Reading

Schuur, J.D., and A.K. Venkatesh. "The Growing Role of Emergency Departments in Hospital Admissions." *New England Journal of Medicine* 367, no. 5 (2012): 391–93.

Chapter 15
Self-Inflicted Injuries

Barry C.L., S.E. Gollust, and J. Niederdeppe. "Are Americans Ready to Solve the Weight of the Nation?" *New England Journal of Medicine* 367, no. 5 (2012): 389–91.

Ghandehari, E., et al. "Abdominal Obesity and the Spectrum of Global Cardiometabolic Risks in US Adults." *Int J Obesity* 33, no. 2(2009): 239–48.

Ogden, C.L., et al. "Prevalence in High Body Mass Index in US Children and Adolescents, 2007–2008." *Journal of the American Medical Association* 307, no. 5 (2010): 483–90.

Further Reading

Barry, C.L., S.E. Gollust, and J. Niederdeppe. "Are Americans Ready to Solve the Weight of the Nation?" *New England Journal of Medicine* 367, no. 5 (2012): 389–91.

Biagi, E., et al. "Through Ageing, and Beyond: Gut Microbiota and Inflammatory Status in Seniors and Centenarians." PLoS One 5, no. 5 (2010).

Block, G. "Foods Contributing to Energy Intake in the US: Data from NHANES III and NHANES 1999–2000." *J Food Comp Anal* (2004).

Caprio, S. "Calories from Soft Drinks—Do They Matter?" *New England Journal of Medicine* 367, no. 15 (2012): 1462–63.

de Ruyter, J.C., et al. "A Trial of Sugar-Free or Sugar-Sweetened Beverages and Body Weight in Children." *New England Journal of Medicine* 367, no. 15 (2012): 1397–406.

Le, M.T., et al. "Effects of High-Fructose Corn Syrup and Sucrose on the Pharmacokinectics and Acute Metabolic and Hemodynamic Responses in Healthy Subjects. *Metabolism* (May 2012).

Lozupone, C.A., et al. "Diversity, Stability, and Resilience of the Human Gut Microbiota." *Nature* 489, no. 7415 (2012): 220–30.

Qi, Q., et al. "Sugar-Sweetened Beverages and Genetic Risk of Obesity." *New England Journal of Medicine* 367, no. 15 (2012): 1387–96.

Qin, J., et al. "A Metagenome-Wide Association Study of Gut Microbiota in Type 2 Diabetes." *Nature* 490, no. 7418 (2012): 55–60.

Chapter 16
It's What You Need to Know, Not What You Want to Know

Scheinhorn, D.J., et al. "Ventilator-Dependent Survivors of Catastrophic Illness Transferred to 23 Long-Term Care Hospitals for Weaning from Prolonged Mechanical Ventilation." *Chest* 131, no. 1 (2007): 76–84.

Kahn, J.M., et al. "Long-Term Acute Care Hospitals Utilization after Critical Illness." *Journal of the American Medical Association* 303, no. 22 (2010): 2253–59.

Grynbaum, M. " Bloomberg Plans a Ban on Large Sugared Drinks."*The New York Times*, May 30, 2012.

Chapter 17
Public and Not-So-Public Debates about Health Care

Chapter 18
The Mystical Wisdom of the Market

Heffner, A.C., et al. "Regionalization of Post-Cardiac Arrest Care: Implementation of a Cardiac Resuscitation Center. *American Heart Journal* 164, no. 4 (2012): 493–501 e2.

Neubauer, S. "The Failing Heart—An Engine Out of Fuel." *New England Journal of Medicine* 356, no. 11 (2007): 1140–51.

Reuben, D.B., and M.E. Tinetti. "Goal-Oriented Patient Care—An Alternative Health Outcomes Paradigm." *New England Journal of Medicine* 366, no. 9 (2012): 777–79.

Further Reading

Robinton, D.A., and G.Q. Daley. "The Promise of Induced Pluripotent Stem Cells in Research and Therapy." *Nature* 481, no. 7381 (2012): 295–305.

Chapter 19
Crafty Intuition, Slim Evidence, and Strong Convictions

Brower, R.G., and J.T. Sylvester. "Solbert Permutt, MD. March 6, 1925–May 23, 2012." *Amer J Resp Crit Care Med* (2012).

DeVita, V.T., and S.A. Rosenberg. "Two Hundred Years of Cancer Research." *New England Journal of Medicine* 366, no. 23 (2012): 2207–14.

Takahashi, K., and S. Yamanaka S. "Induction of Pluripotent Stem Cells from Mouse Embryonic and Adult Fibroblast Cultures by Defined Factors." *Cell* 126, no. 4 (2006): 663–76.

Further Reading

Curtis, C., et al. "The Genomic and Transcriptomic Architecture of 2,000 Breast Tumours Reveals Novel Subgroups." *Nature* 486, no. 7403 (2012): 346–52.

Ellis, M.J., et al. "Whole-Genome Analysis Informs Breast Cancer Response to Aromatase Inhibition." *Nature* 486, no. 7403 (2012): 353–60.

Qian, L., et al. "In Vivo Reprogramming of Murine Cardiac Fibroblasts into Induced Cardiomyocytes." *Nature* 485, no. 7400 (2012): 593–+.

Chapter 20
Equitable Allocation of Finite Services

Gupta, S. "More Treatment, More Mistakes." *The New York Times*, July 2012.

Lembke, A. "Why Doctors Prescribe Opoids to Known Opoid Abusers." *New England Journal of Medicine 367,no.17* (2012) 1580-1.

Rosenbaum, L., and D. Laurus. "Cents and Sensitivity—Teaching Physicians to Think about Costs." *New England Journal of Medicine* (2012).

Stevens, R. "Goodbye, Bicentennial: The Recurrent Crisis of Medical Education." *New England Journal of Medicine* (295,no.25 1(976) 1252-54.

Further Reading

Sommers, B.D., K. Baicker, and A.M. Epstein, "Mortality and Access to Care among Adults after State Medicaid Expansions." *New England Journal of Medicine* 367, no. 11 (2012): 1025–34.

Chapter 21
Disadvantaged and Worse

Joshi, S., et al. "Review of Ethnic Disparities in Access to Renal Transplantation." *Clinical Transplantation* (2012).

Kimball, M.M., et al. "Race and Income Disparity in Ischemic Stroke Care: Nationwide Inpatient Sample Database, 2002–2008." *J Stroke Cerebrovasc Dis* ,July 17,(2012).

LoConte, N.K., et al. "Increasing Disparity in Colorectal Cancer Incidence and Mortality among African Americans and Whites: A State's Experience." *J Gastrointest. Oncology* 2, no.2(2011) 85-92.

Silver, R.M., et al. "Racial Differences between Blacks and Whites with Systemic Sclerosis." *Curr Opin Rheumatol* (2012).

Further Reading

Kellermann, A.L. and R.M. Weinick. "Emergency Departments, Medicaid Costs, and Access to Primary Care—Understanding the Link. New England Journal of Medicine ,366,no23(2012) 2141-43.

Zheng, L., et al. "Lung Cancer Survival among Black and White Patients in an Equal Access Health System." *Cancer Epidemiol Biomarkers Prev* 21, no. 10 (2012): 1841–7.

Chapter 22
Profitable Networking—Is It Profitable to Treat This Condition?

Further Reading

Bernstein, N. "Hospitals Flout Charity Aid Law." *The New York Times*, February 2012.

Neumann, P.J. "What We Talk about When We Talk about Health Care Costs." *New England Journal of Medicine* 366, no. 7 (2012): 585–586.

Chapter 23
A Conversation with Dr. Sharon Rounds

Trivedi, A., et al. "Comparison of the Quality of Medical Care in Veterans Affairs and Non-Veterans Affairs Settings." *Medical Care* (January 2011).

Chapter 24
Medical Care in the Netherlands—A Model for US Reform?

Chapter 25
Big and Not-So-Big Pharma

Chapter 26
A Virtual Conversation about the Prospects of Health Care Reform in America

Forrest, C.B. "Strengthening Primary Care to Bolster the Health Care Safety Net." *Journal of the American Medical Association* 295, no. 9 (2006): 1062–64.

Marmot, M. "Status Syndrome: A Challenge to Medicine." *Journal of the American Medical Association* 295, no. 11 (2006): 1304–07.

Further Reading

Barnes, K.A., J.C. Kroening–Roche, and B.W. Comfort. "Becoming a Physician: The Developing Vision of Primary Care." *New England Journal of Medicine* 367, no. 10 (2012): 891–93.

Scott, A., et al. "The Effect of Financial Incentives on the Quality of Health Care Provided by Primary Care Physicians." Cochrane Database Syst Rev (2011).

Chapter 27
Recommendations for Baby Boomers

Further Reading

Fritsch, T., et al. "Cognitive Functioning in Healthy Aging: The Role of Reserve and Lifestyle Factors Early in Life." *Gerontologist* 47, no. 3 (2007): 307–22.

"Simple Treatments, Ignored." *The New York Times*, September 2012.

Schwartz, J. "Logging On for a Second (or Third) Opinion." *The New York Times*, September 2008.

www.ingramcontent.com/pod-product-compliance
Lightning Source LLC
Chambersburg PA
CBHW040125270326
41926CB00001B/12